D1212842

Practical Echocardiography of Congenital Heart Disease

MCP HAHNEMANN UNIVERSITY
HAHNEMANN LIBRARY

Practical Echocardiography of Congenital Heart Disease

From Fetus to Adult

David T. Linker, M.D.
Associate Professor of Medicine
Division of Cardiology
University of Washington School of Medicine
Co-Director, Adult Congenital Heart Disease Clinic
Associate Director, Echocardiography Laboratory
University of Washington Medical Center
Seattle, Washington

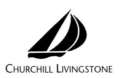

CHURCHILL LIVINGSTONE

A Harcourt Health Sciences Company
New York   Edinburgh   London   Philadelphia

CHURCHILL LIVINGSTONE
A Harcourt Health Sciences Company

The Curtis Center
Independence Square West
Philadelphia, Pennsylvania 19106

Library of Congress Cataloging-in-Publication Data

Linker, David T.
Practical echocardiography of congenital heart disease: from fetus to adult / David T.
Linker.—Ed. 1.

p.   cm.

ISBN 0–443–07640–5

1. Congenital heart disease—Diagnosis.   2. Echocardiography.   I. Title.
[DNLM: 1. Heart Defects, Congenital—ultrasonography.   2. Echocardiography—
methods.   3. Heart Defects, Congenital—embryology. WG 220 L756e 2001]

RC687.L56 2001   616.1′2043—dc21   00–064372

Acquisitions Editor: Marc Strauss
Project Manager: Agnes Hunt Byrne
Production Manager: Norman Stellander
Illustration Specialist: Lisa Lambert
Indexer: Dennis Dolan

PRACTICAL ECHOCARDIOGRAPHY OF CONGENITAL HEART DISEASE   ISBN 0–443–07640–5

Copyright © 2001 by Churchill Livingstone.

All rights reserved. No part of this publication may be reproduced or transmitted in any form or by any means, electronic or mechanical, including photocopy, recording, or any information storage and retrieval system, without permission in writing from the publisher.

Churchill Livingstone and the Sail Boat Design are trademarks of Harcourt, Inc., registered in the United States of America and/or other jurisdictions.

Printed in the United States of America.

Last digit is the print number: 9   8   7   6   5   4   3   2   1

To my parents, Hal and Halla Linker,
with love and deep appreciation
for the priceless gifts they have given me

Features of This Book

● Practical orientation
● Organized by age and presenting symptom and sign
● Severity evaluation as well as diagnosis
● Most illustration sequences are from a single patient
● Both pediatric and adult orientation of views
● Echocardiographic images do not have structures labeled
● Boxed lists for:
   Screening examination
   Potential diagnoses
   Potential findings
   Sufficient examination

Preface

Any good preface should at least answer the question of why the reader should read this book. I believe the best answer is: This is the book I wanted when I was starting out.

There are many good books on echocardiography and even many on echocardiography of congenital heart disease. What distinguishes this book from the others is a strong emphasis on the practical (see Box). The spectrum of potential diagnoses varies greatly, depending on the age group being examined, and the presenting problem determines what the diagnoses should explain. For this reason, most of the chapters deal with a specific age group and are organized by presenting problem. In addition to pointing out the details to look for in a particular diagnosis, there is also an emphasis on what is sufficient to make a congenital heart defect extremely unlikely as the cause of the presenting problem for a patient in that age group.

This means that the thrust is to think of echocardiography as a tool to solve clinical problems. The particular problem depends first on the clinical presentation and age of the patient, but once we have made a diagnosis, there is also the issue of determining the severity of the diagnosis. For this reason, most of the figures are not simply a single "good illustration," but rather they are a sequence of images taken from a single patient with the problem being demonstrated, showing not only the features necessary for diagnosis but also the factors necessary to determine severity. The images do not have structures labeled, since the images used for diagnosis do not come with labels attached. Where the features may be difficult to identify, a line drawing has been created to show the anatomic details.

The intended audience is both those who are new to the field of echocardiography or congenital heart disease, and those who are experienced in other areas of echocardiography but deal with congenital heart disease infrequently. This is not intended to be an encyclopedic text for the center specializing in congenital heart disease. Because of this, many rare and complex problems are either mentioned only briefly or not at all, and the very complex topic of follow-up of patients with complex repairs is touched on only lightly.

In spite of this, this book can stand on its own as a "first text," or a "practical guide." Chapter 1 details the principles behind echocardiographic imaging, and Chapter 2 gives an anatomic and physiological framework for understanding congenital heart disease. Chapters 3 to 6 deal with different age groups: fetus, newborn and infant, toddler and child, and finally teenager and adult. There are two appendices, covering standard echocardiographic views and the complex topic of heterotaxy, and a bibliography.

For each age group, there is a summary of what one can find on the screening examination. For each of the age groups and presenting problems, there are lists of what the most likely potential diagnoses and echocardiographic findings are, as well as what findings would constitute sufficient negative evidence for congenital heart disease being an explanation of the clinical problem.

I was trained in both adult and pediatric cardiology in the United States, but have practiced in Norway and the Netherlands as well. In Norway, the echocardiographic studies are performed by the cardiologists as part of the clinic visit or inpatient consultation. Most of the echocardiographic images were collected by me in this manner and recorded on VHS tape. Most of the images in Chapter 6 were acquired by the sonographers at the University of Washington Medical Center Echocardiography Laboratory and were recorded on S-VHS tape.

The images were digitized directly from the videotape using either a Macintosh Quadra 800, or 8100/80 AV with Radius Video Vision Studio hardware. The other hardware used was a Macintosh "Blue and White" G3 with Aurora Fuse video card. The images digitized from VHS tape were stabilized by using a FERAL time base corrector/synchronizer before digitization. All of the digitized images were processed in Adobe Photoshop, with some correction for contrast and digitization artifacts. Some of the images in Chapter 3 were photographed directly from the screen.

The line drawings were mostly made with Macromedia FreeHand version 7.0, by me. The exceptions are Figures 2–1, 2–2A, 2–10, 4–12A and B, which were drawn by Starr Kaplan expressly for this book, and Figures A–1, A–2, A–6, A–8, and A–9, which are used with permission from the American Society of Echocardiography. These images were digitized from the original publication at 400 DPI using a Visioneer PaperPort Vx scanner and the resulting images were enhanced in Photoshop.

DAVID THOR LINKER, M.D.

Acknowledgments

Any work has a number of contributors, both direct and indirect. This book is no exception. Although most of the images used in this book were collected by me, some were created by the excellent sonographers in the echocardiography laboratory at the University of Washington Medical Center, including Carolyn Miyake-Hull, Carol Kraft, Michelle Fujioka, Rebecca Schwaegler, Todd Zwink, Scott Simicich, and Carolyn Gardner. Some of the images in Chapters 4 and 5 were created by Dr. Wendy Williams, who was in training in pediatric cardiology at the time.

A number of people have helped by reading the preliminary text. Foremost among these is Dr. Warren Guntheroth, who has taken the brunt, reading every chapter. Any errors or omissions that remain in the text are probably due to my not following his generous and well-founded advice. Others who have read chapters and provided useful comments are Drs. Brad Munt and Stephanie Cooper, and sonographers Carol Kraft and Carolyn Miyake-Hull.

I also owe a great debt to those who taught me echocardiography. As Newton said, "If I have seen farther, it is by standing on the shoulders of giants." Drs. Alan Pearlman, Richard Popp, and Liv Hatle contributed greatly to my understanding of the principles and practice of echocardiography.

Expert secretarial help was provided by Stephanie Kruzan and Kay Schmidt.

My family has also supported this effort. My thanks go to my wife, Margaret, who understood the importance of the time spent on completing this book, and my son Matthew, who had trouble understanding why his father didn't always have time to do "guy things" together on the weekend.

My greatest debt is to my parents, Hal and Halla Linker. Not only did they always give me love and support, but they also gave me the foundation of critical thinking and care for others that led me to and have served me well in a career in medicine.

Contents

Practical
Echocardiography
of
Congenital
Heart Disease

Color Plates

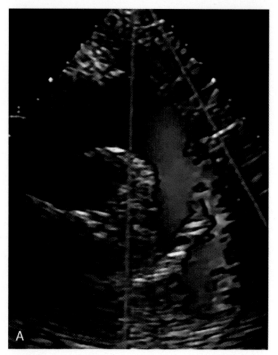

Figure 1–17. Reflection can also affect Doppler signals. *A*, in a suprasternal view of the aortic arch, it is possible to see the color flow in the descending aorta. There also appears to be color flow exiting from the aorta and is even visible in a "channel" located posterior to the aorta.

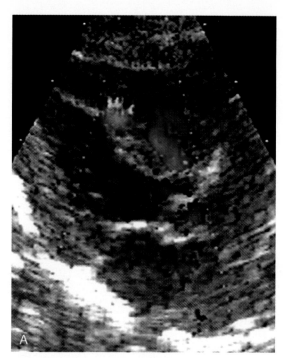

Figure 4–3. *A*, A parasternal long-axis view of the color flow through a small to moderate muscular ventricular septal defect in a 5-day-old newborn.

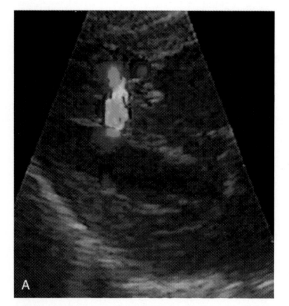

Figure 4–5. *A*, A parasternal long-axis view of flow through a moderate-sized muscular ventricular septal defect in a 2-day-old newborn.

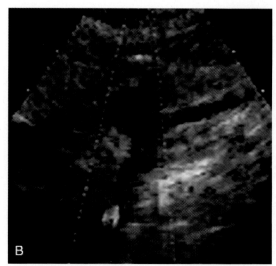

Figure 4–6. Image from a 10-day-old infant presenting with difficulty feeding. *B*, The color Doppler of the descending aorta, which has a small area of disturbed flow as shown by the green coloration.

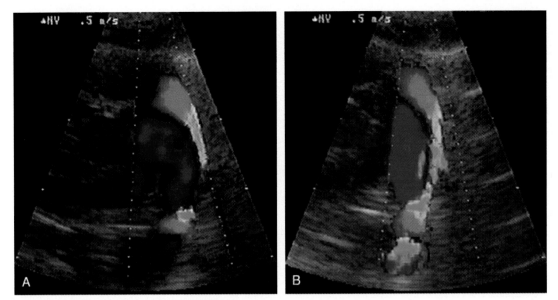

Figure 4–7. *A,* A color Doppler parasternal short-axis view of the pulmonary artery (blue) and its branches as well as the reverse-flow jet through a patent ductus arteriosus. This newborn was 2 days old at the time and had an asymptomatic continuous murmur. Note the location of the jet relative to the pulmonary artery branches. It is overlying the left pulmonary artery, because the ductus is actually to the left and superior to the left pulmonary artery. *B,* The same ductal flow at a slightly different time in the cardiac cycle, showing how markedly different the color can look for the same physiology.

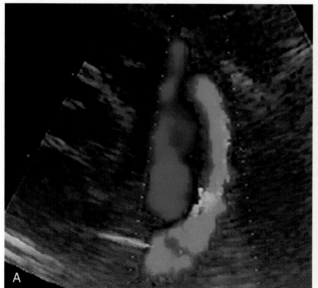

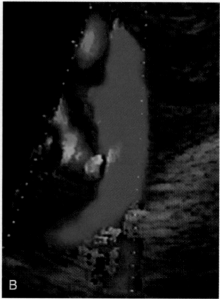

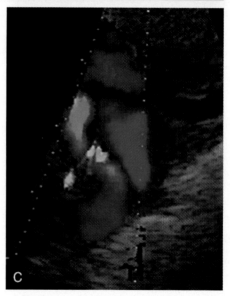

Figure 4–11. Another indication of hemodynamic significance for a patent ductus arteriosus is flow reversal in the descending aorta. *A*, A parasternal short-axis view of the color flow of a nonrestrictive ductus arteriosus, demonstrated by the lack of evidence for flow acceleration or turbulence. *B*, A suprasternal view of the aortic arch, with anterograde flow in the descending aorta (blue) and retrograde flow (red) in the ductus arteriosus during systole. *C*, The same view in diastole, with retrograde flow (red) from the descending aorta distal to the ductus, into the ductus.

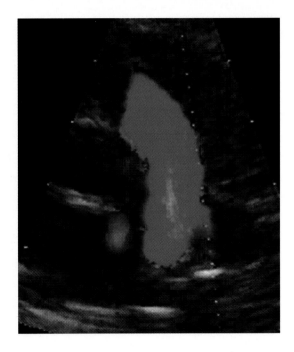

Figure 4–16. Parasternal view of the normal crossing of the pulmonary artery and the aorta in a 2-month-old. The pulmonary artery flow is visible as blue, flowing away from the transducer toward the lungs. The aorta is visible running from the midportion on the left down and to the right. Note how the two arteries cross almost perpendicularly.

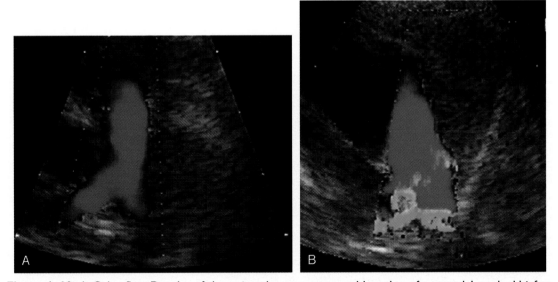

Figure 4–19. A, Color flow Doppler of the main pulmonary artery and branches of a normal 1-week-old infant. Note that there is no disturbed flow. B, The color flow Doppler of the main pulmonary artery and branches of a 1-month-old infant with a systolic murmur radiating to the lungs. There is disturbed flow at both of the branch points.

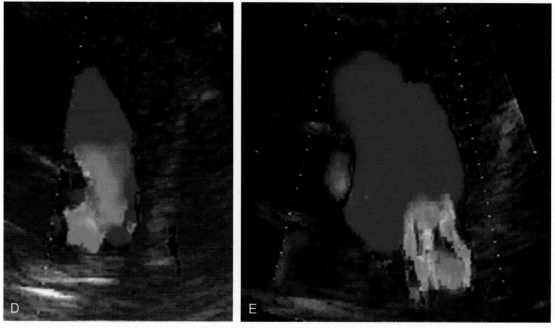

Figure 4–19 *Continued.* This is the result of a normal variant, with relative narrowing of the origin of the right and left pulmonary arteries, and this is a functional pulmonary flow murmur. It does not always affect both sides. It can affect only the right *(D)* or the left side *(E)*.

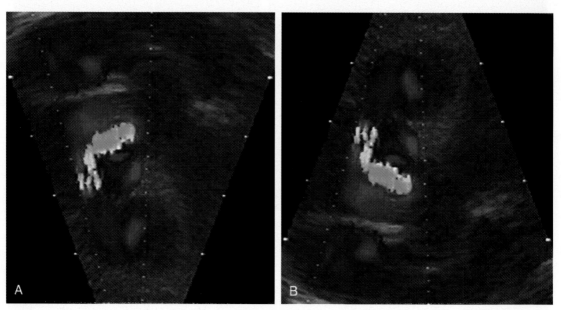

Figure 4–20. *A,* An apical 5-chamber view of the flow through a small membranous ventricular septal defect in a 6-week-old infant with a murmur ("pediatric" orientation). *B,* The same image in the "adult" orientation.

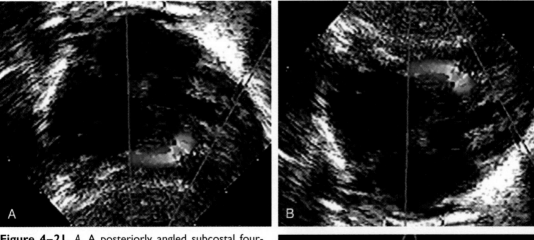

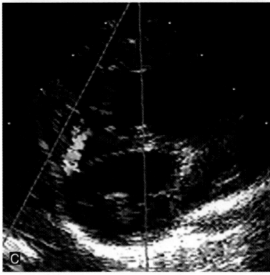

Figure 4–21. A, A posteriorly angled subcostal four-chamber view taken from a newborn with a systolic murmur (standard "pediatric" orientation). B, The same image in the "adult" orientation. There is evidence of disturbed flow across the ventricular septum, from the left to the right ventricle. C, The short-axis view on the same patient demonstrating the posterior location of the small muscular ventricular septal defect.

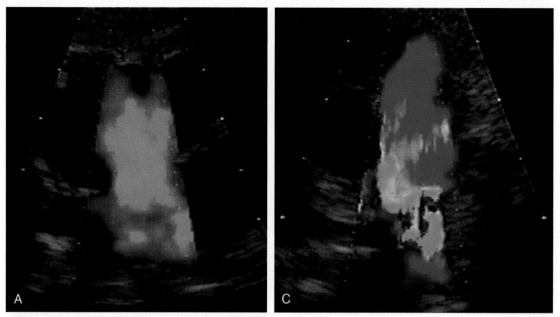

Figure 4–25. These images are from a 7-month-old infant with a murmur. *A,* A subcostal four-chamber view with definite color Doppler flow across the interatrial septum, from the left atrium to the right atrium. *C,* The murmur came from the increased and disturbed pulmonic flow, as shown in the parasternal short-axis color flow image.

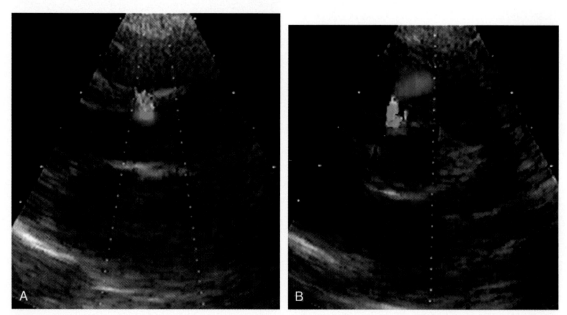

Figure 5–2. *A,* The color flow image from the parasternal long-axis view in a 2½-year-old with an asymptomatic murmur. There is evidence for left-to-right flow through a small perimembranous ventricular septal defect, just below the aortic valve. *B,* The same ventricular septal defect from the short-axis view. Note the tricuspid valve visible just to the left of the color flow.

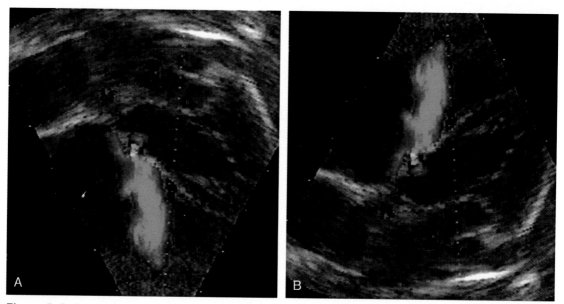

Figure 5–3. Images from a 9-month-old with an asymptomatic systolic murmur. *A,* A subcostal four-chamber view taken with the transducer moved laterally from the midline and the image oriented in the pediatric view. It shows the flow through a restrictive ventricular septal defect in the perimembranous position. *B,* The same image in the adult orientation.

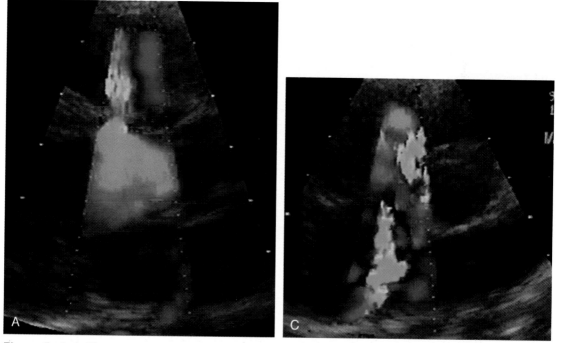

Figure 5–4. *A,* The parasternal long-axis view of the heart of a 13-month-old with an asymptomatic systolic murmur. There is flow from the left ventricle to the right ventricle across a perimembranous ventricular septal defect. Note that this image does not show disturbed flow, which raises the question of elevation of the right-sided pressures, or a false-positive color flow image. *C,* The short-axis parasternal view, with the relationship of the ventricular septal defect flow and the tricuspid regurgitation.

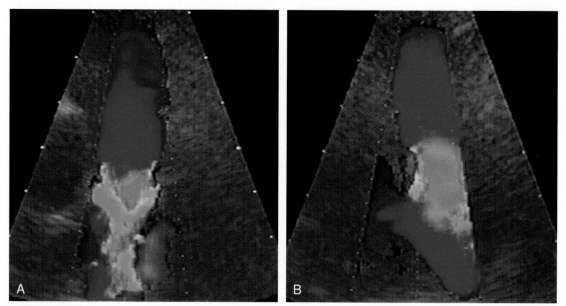

Figure 5–5. A 5-year-old child with a pulmonary systolic murmur. *A,* The color flow through the pulmonary outflow from the parasternal short-axis view. Note the disturbed (green) flow. This could be pulmonic stenosis or atrial septal defect or a normal variant. *B,* At other times in the cardiac cycle, the flow is not disturbed but does exceed the velocity-aliasing limit, changing color to red.

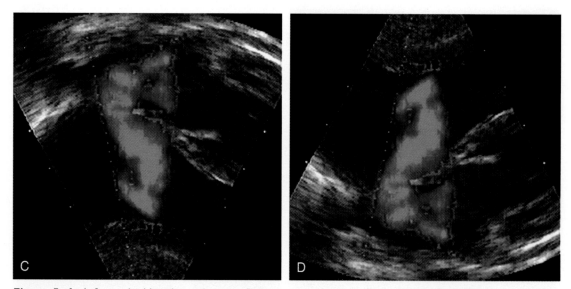

Figure 5–6. A 9-month-old with a pulmonary flow murmur. *C* and *D,* The subcostal four-chamber view in the standard pediatric and adult orientations, respectively, demonstrating color flow across the interatrial septum, from the left atrium to right atrium.

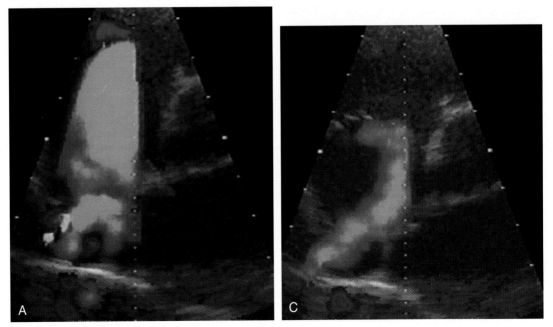

Figure 5–7. Images from a 6-year-old with an asymptomatic murmur. The parasternal short-axis view of the atrial septum with color looks like a secundum atrial septal defect *(A)*. In fact, this is flow from the inferior vena cava. *C*, A slight change in angle shows the flow coming from the inferior vena cava.

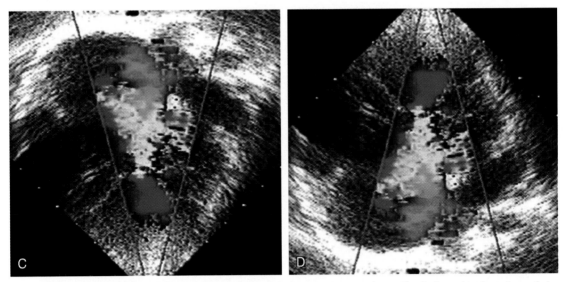

Figure 5–11. *C* and *D*, The standard pediatric and adult orientations of an off-axis four-chamber view of the same child (as in *A* and *B*), demonstrating significant color flow coming from a left ventricular to right atrial shunt. Note that the tricuspid valve to the left of the color sector is not the source of the disturbed flow.

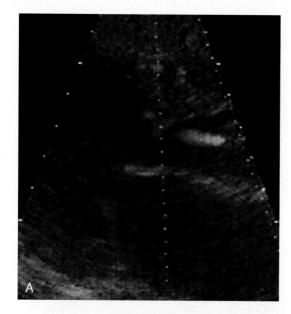

Figure 5–12. *A,* The color Doppler of aortic insufficiency in an 18-year-old who has an asymptomatic diastolic murmur. The view is a parasternal long axis, and a small jet of aortic insufficiency is visible.

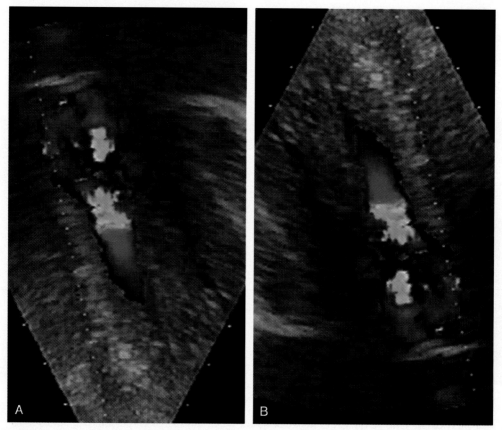

Figure 5–13. These color images are from the same child as in Figure 5–8 and are the same image, shown in different orientations. *A,* The pediatric orientation. *B,* The adult orientation. Each is a color Doppler of the left ventricular outflow tract taken from the apical position. Note the disturbed flow in the left ventricular outflow tract.

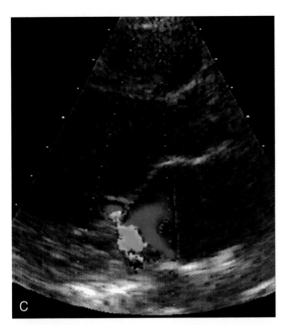

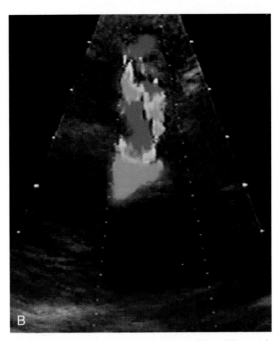

Figure 5–14. Images from an 8-year-old girl who presented with decreased exercise tolerance. *C*, Shows mitral regurgitation by color Doppler.

Figure 5–15. Image from a 1-year-old toddler with tetralogy of Fallot. *B*, The flow across the defect from left to right, which is low velocity because the defect is not restrictive.

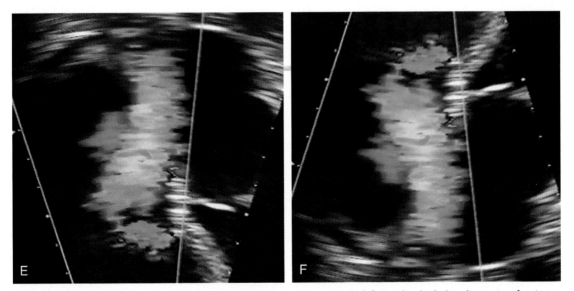

Figure 6–3. Images from a patient with an atrial secundum septal defect who had the diagnosis of primary pulmonary hypertension before this echo was performed. *E*, The flow through the atrial septal defect, from a view intermediate between an apical and subcostal view, in the pediatric orientation. *F*, The same image in the adult orientation.

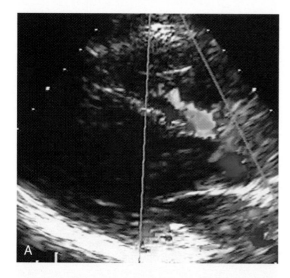

Figure 6–4. Image from a patient with an asymptomatic murmur since childhood. *A,* A long-axis view demonstrating systolic flow across the membranous portion of the ventricular septum.

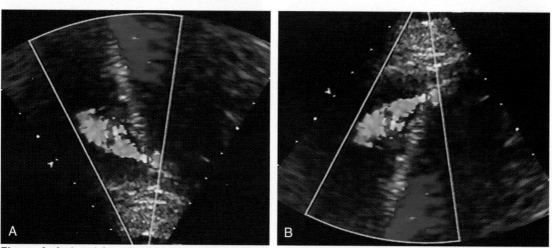

Figure 6–6. Apical four-chamber view in a patient with an asymptomatic murmur. There is clear shunting from the left ventricle to the right ventricle in the apex on the four-chamber, zoomed view (*A,* pediatric orientation; *B,* adult orientation).

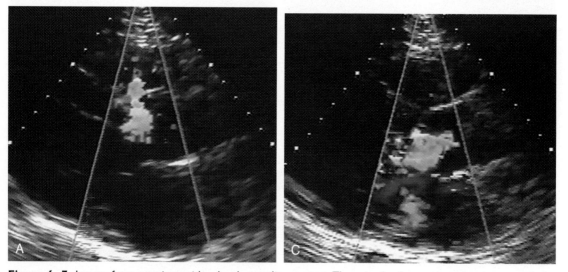

Figure 6–7. Images from a patient with a harsh systolic murmur. There is clearly a perimembranous ventricular septal defect *(A),* which is restrictive. There is also aortic insufficiency *(C).*

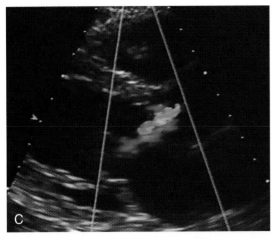

Figure 6–8. Image from a patient with an asymptomatic murmur from a bicuspid aortic valve. *C*, Mild aortic regurgitation, which is common.

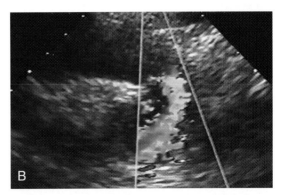

Figure 6–10. Image from a patient with hypertension and a murmur. *B*, There is acceleration of flow in the abnormal region in the descending aortic arch.

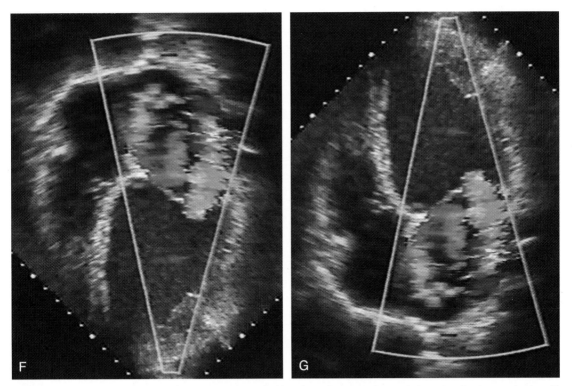

Figure 6–13. These images are from a patient with dilated cardiomyopathy, and there is mitral regurgitation (*F*, pediatric orientation; *G*, adult orientation).

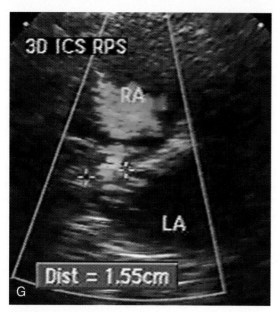

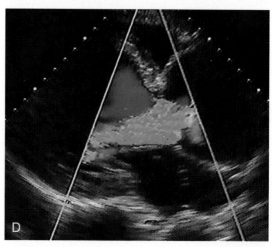

Figure 6–15. This patient had murmur and decreased exercise tolerance. From an unusual location, it was possible to demonstrate flow across a sinus venosus atrial septal defect with color flow (G).

Figure 6–18. Images from a patient with Marfan syndrome who presented with back pain and symptoms of congestive heart failure. There is aortic insufficiency (D), which causes end-diastolic flow reversal in the abdominal aorta.

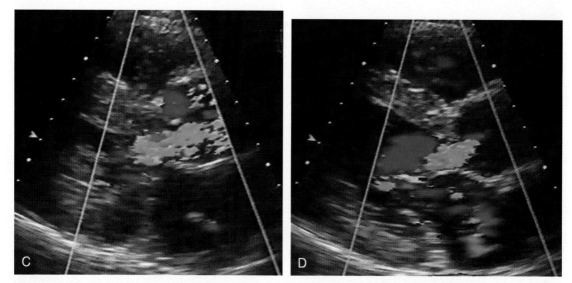

Figure 6–19. This patient has a subaortic membrane with a significant gradient. Color flow mapping shows both the flow acceleration through the membrane (C) and the aortic insufficiency (D), which is common in this condition.

Introduction

The Clinical Presentation

All useful textbooks have some organizing principle, which establishes both the order of presentation and the logical sequence. Most textbooks of echocardiography are organized based on the patient's diagnosis or specific ultrasound technique used or some combination of the two. These are powerful principles, which lead to clear categories and little duplication. When a patient presents in the clinic or on the ward, however, symptoms and signs predominate. Few patients present with a complete diagnosis or for a specific type of examination. Fortunately, the signs and symptoms generally fall into recognizable patterns, referred to as clinical presentations, and these are actually fewer in number than potential diagnoses. These clinical presentations, therefore, can provide a different type of organizing principle.

The beginner in echocardiography needs a guide to help with the step from the clinical presentations of disease to the precise diagnosis and evaluation of a disease. This book is intended as an aid in the evaluation of congenital heart disease when an ultrasonic examination is performed. Patients do not arrive in the echocardiography laboratory with a blank slate. We always know something about the patient's age, and this rather severely alters the spectrum of potential disease. It seems appropriate to give this information an early position in our evaluation scheme. In addition, the patient is referred to examination because a particular set of signs and symptoms may suggest disease or for evaluation of a known defect. This can provide the next level of division in our evaluation. In either case, one can conceptually divide the evaluation into definition of the anatomy and quantification of the physiology. In addition, we can divide the assessment of the lesion into the primary findings associated with the defect, the secondary effects, which are a result of the lesion, and finally, related lesions, which can also have their own primary and secondary findings (Box 1–1).

As an example, we can take the clinical presentation of an asymptomatic older child with a coarse systolic murmur at the right upper sternal border, radiating to the neck. In this case, the clinical problem is possible aortic stenosis, or bicuspid aortic valve. For our primary anatomic evaluation, we would examine the aortic valve, looking at the number and shape of the leaflets as well as their mobility. For our primary physiological evaluation, we would use continuous-wave or high pulse repetition frequency (PRF) Doppler to evaluate the velocity across the valve and calculate the gradient. Secondary anatomic changes would include poststenotic dilation of the ascending aorta and increased thickness of the left ventricle. Secondary physiological changes would include alterations in the mitral diastolic flow pattern, reflecting abnormal filling of the left ventricle. Finally, we know that aortic stenosis is often associated with aortic regurgitation, so we would use Doppler to detect and quantitate any leakage (Box 1–2).

BOX 1–1
ELEMENTS OF A COMPLETE EVALUATION

Anatomy
  Primary—main diagnosis
  Secondary—expected anatomic consequences
  Related—other diagnoses that may be present
Physiology
  Primary—severity
  Secondary—expected physiological consequences
  Related—physiology of other diagnoses

BOX 1–2
ELEMENTS OF EVALUATION OF
VALVULAR AORTIC STENOSIS

Anatomy

Primary—mobility, thickness, number of
leaflets

Secondary—poststenotic dilation of aorta,
left ventricular hypertrophy, or dilation

Related—subvalvular narrowing, poor
closure (insufficiency)

Physiology

Primary—transvalvular gradient

Secondary—abnormal transmitral flow, left
ventricular dysfunction

Related—subvalvular gradient, aortic
insufficiency

There are several advantages to this sort of approach. The divisions into anatomic/physiological and primary/secondary/related function as a mnemonic aid and reference, helping the examiner to perform a complete examination. Once we have performed such an examination, we can evaluate the severity of the lesion in addition to the diagnosis. Finally, we can improve the accuracy of our diagnoses by this approach, because the presence of the entire constellation of anatomic/physiological, primary/secondary findings strongly supports the diagnosis, whereas absence of expected findings in the constellation may reduce the degree of certainty.

A disadvantage of the approach taken in this book is that a given concept or disease entity may logically fall into several age groups or clinical presentations. This will lead to a certain amount of repetition and cross-referencing. In general, if the situation is virtually identical to that discussed in another section of the book, there will be a brief discussion and reference to the other section. If there are significant differences, the subject will be discussed in each section that it is necessary.

In clinical medicine, we are constantly reminded that ours is an applied science, with an emphasis on solutions to practical problems as opposed to understanding for

knowledge's sake. I hope that this book will help provide a bridge from the technical details of the clinical echocardiographic examination to the practical world of clinical problem solving.

THE INTEGRATED EXAMINATION

When we perform an echocardiographic examination, our goal must be to answer the clinical questions as accurately as possible. Whether we use two-dimensional imaging or pulsed Doppler is not important except as it affects the sensitivity and specificity of our examination. Each technique has its own drawbacks and advantages with respect to a given type of examination, and in many cases we must integrate the results of several different type of examination to come to a complete understanding of the anatomy and physiology.

If an integrated examination leads to a complete understanding, it follows that lack of integration must lead to incomplete understanding. All of us have a tendency to become more proficient with certain techniques than with others. Overreliance on a few of the available methods must lead to a reduction in our diagnostic accuracy or sensitivity. This conclusion underscores the importance of sharpening our skills in all of the echocardiographic modalities and using the strengths of one to offset the deficiencies of the others.

The principles underlying each of the main techniques of the echocardiographic examination determine the strengths and weaknesses of the technique. By understanding the generation of the signals we will interpret, we can also understand the potential sources of error or misinterpretation.

Imaging

Echocardiographic imaging is based on reflected ultrasound, using techniques borrowed from sonar and radar. Ultrasound is sound at a frequency well above the range audible to humans and is defined as any

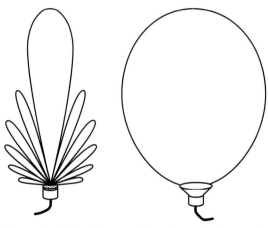

Figure 1–1. The direction of maximum signal strength for the ultrasound transducer is called the beam *(left)* and is highly focused compared with the sound coming out of a loudspeaker *(right)*. The reason for this is that the wavelength of the ultrasound is short compared with the width of the transducer, whereas the wavelength of the sound coming out of the speaker is long compared with the width of the speaker. The width of the beam is inversely proportional to the product of frequency times the width of the transducer. Note also the lobes of sensitivity directed to the side of the main lobe, exaggerated here for illustration. These are called side lobes and are the cause of some "false" echo images, discussed later in this chapter.

sound with a frequency greater than 20,000 cycles per second, or 20 kHz. Most diagnostic ultrasound uses frequencies from 2 to 10 MHz (or million cycles per second). At the high frequencies of sound used for diagnostic cardiac studies, the sound energy is highly focused, and the distribution resembles the beam of a flashlight more than the sound coming from a loudspeaker (Fig. 1–1). Because the wavelength of the sound is similar in dimension to the size of the transducer, there are diffraction effects, causing peaks and valleys in the transmitted signal strength and also in the reception sensitivity. This is an important detail that is discussed in further detail later (see Pitfalls and Artifacts).

The basic principle of ultrasound imaging is similar to that of sonar. A pulse of sound is transmitted, and returning echoes are recorded as amplitude as a function of time. A returning echo is generated whenever the ultrasound energy encounters a change in sound transmission properties, which are determined by the density and compressibility of the tissue. It is important to remember that it is changes in the properties, not absolute values of the properties, that generate a reflection. Blood plasma alone would not generate any reflection, whereas an interface between plasma and muscle would because of the change in properties.

The frequency used has many important effects. First, the focusing becomes sharper as the frequency becomes higher because of the narrowing of the beam. Second, the resolution along the beam becomes higher because the wavelength becomes shorter. The wavelength defines the theoretical lower limit of resolution, whereas the pulse is usually a given number of wavelengths long, regardless of the actual wavelength. The pulse length determines the actual resolution limit, because even a sharp interface will create an echo which is a reflection of the outgoing pulse. Third, the rate at which the ultrasound energy becomes weaker with depth becomes more rapid at higher frequencies. There is also a decrease in the maximum velocity that can be correctly identified with Doppler, which is discussed later (see Doppler).

The practical consequences of these factors are that, for imaging, we generally want to use the highest frequency possible but are often limited by the poorer ultrasound penetration at higher frequencies. If ultrasound penetration is poor, we want to decrease the frequency of the ultrasound we are using for imaging. For Doppler, we are generally not as interested in high resolution, so lower frequencies are beneficial for both better penetration and higher velocity limits (Box 1–3).

BOX 1–3
EFFECTS OF INCREASED FREQUENCY

Improved lateral resolution

Improved axial resolution

Decreased penetration

Lower Doppler velocity limit

Two-Dimensional Imaging

To generate a two-dimensional cross-section, we need to cause the flashlight-like beam to point in different directions. In each direction, the ultrasound instrument sends out a pulse of ultrasound and records the resulting echoes. Typically, 128 or more such "beams" are used to create each cross-sectional image. The simplest way to understand how the beam can be moved is with a mechanical motion of the transducer, so that it points in various directions (Fig. 1–2). This can be either a rotation or a wobbling motion. Systems based on this principle have the advantage of having a symmetric beam, which is the same in all directions. The major disadvantage is that the system is mechanical and may break down.

Another method that has increasingly gained popularity is to use an array of very small transducers and to control the relative time of excitation of the transducers. By gradually delaying the time of excitation, the effective wave front will be pointed in a direction off of the main axis of the transducer. Using a similar technique and delaying the received signals, the effective maximum sensitivity to receive a signal can be pointed in different directions. This technique is called a *phased array* and has the advantage of no moving parts. The disadvantage is that the beam is not as narrow

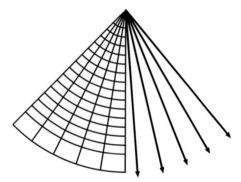

Figure 1–3. Each beam *(right)* is used to generate a set of values for each depth and the angle between it and the adjacent beams *(left)*. The beam data are very dense close to the transducer and very sparse far away. For this reason, interpolation methods are used to improve the appearance of the data in the distant areas. Only a very limited number of beams are illustrated here. The actual number is typically 128 or higher.

as can be achieved with a mechanical system, and its shape varies as a function of the direction.

Either of these types of system can produce good quality echocardiographic images. The actual ultrasound data that are collected are very detailed in the region close to the transducer because all of the beams converge there (Fig. 1–3). It is very sparse far away from the transducer, and the ultrasound machine has to interpolate the data to form a smooth image. Ultrasound machines may differ in the details of how they perform these functions as well as the adjustments available for the alteration of the gray scale. These differences can account for some of the differences in images obtained on different machines.

M-Mode

One of the limitations of two-dimensional imaging is that the frame rate is limited by the time required to send beams in all the directions to create the cross-section. With a frame rate of 25 to 40 per second, some rapid motions can be difficult to identify correctly. This can be resolved if we keep the beam in one direction and display the signals from this one direction as a function of time. Typically, 1000 pulses are sent in this one direction each second. This tech-

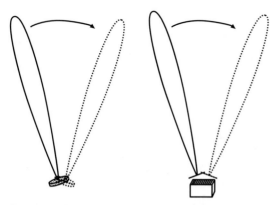

Figure 1–2. The beam can be pointed in different directions either by a mechanical process physically moving the transducer and beam *(left)* or by using an array of small transducers and delaying the activation so that the wave front is effectively pointed in the desired direction *(right)*.

nique is called M-mode (from motion) and is actually much older than two-dimensional imaging.

Any time we want to examine a structure that is moving rapidly, M-mode will give us a more accurate delineation of the motion because of a higher sampling rate. Examples include fetal arrhythmias, valve motion, and identification of vegetations. M-mode also can be easier for measurements in some situations.

Doppler

Doppler echocardiography is the measurement of blood flow velocities to aid in the anatomic diagnosis or physiological evaluation of heart disease. The ability to assess the physiological consequences of heart lesions through the use of Doppler echocardiography has been a major contribution to the utility of echocardiography in general and for congenital heart disease in particu-

lar. Previously, cardiac catheterization was usually required for any assessment of the physiology of defects. This has been almost completely replaced by noninvasive assessment using Doppler techniques.

Doppler echocardiography can, in fact, only measure one parameter: velocity of blood flow. By combining this information with an understanding of the anatomy and the physics of blood flow, we can usually infer the pressure relationships and flow volumes in the heart. As discussed in Chapter 2 (see Physiology), the pressure and flow relationships are central to understanding congenital heart disease.

Measurement of Velocity

Although the principles of Doppler echocardiography can seem confusing, the phenomenon is something we have all experienced, and it can be represented using a simple model, which is accurate in all respects.*

*This basic model of the Doppler effect can be told as a story, which can be understood quite well even by people without a mathematical background. I developed this story as a fellow in pediatric cardiology, when a pleasant secretary in the division asked me to explain the Doppler effect. I took the challenge and chose to incorporate her other major interest outside of her work, which was love stories.

Many hundreds of years ago, in the Middle East, there were two sweethearts who unfortunately lived in different cities. In spite of this, they were able to see each other often because the young man was a successful trader, and, of course, whenever he traveled he made sure that he would visit the city of his sweetheart.

He would let her know that he was coming in one of his daily love letters, which he sent by carrier pigeon, which he used in his successful business as a trader. One of the reasons he was successful was that he was rather precise in all of his transactions, and this carried over to the releasing of the pigeons as well. He always released the pigeon at noon, when the sun was highest in the sky.

His beloved had come to expect the daily arrival of the pigeons and always looked forward to them. She had noted a strange phenomenon, however. When he was on his way to visit her, she found that the pigeons arrived earlier every day. She interpreted this as a sign of his excitement, showing that he had been unable to wait until noon. This pleased her greatly. The real reason was that the pigeons had a shorter distance to fly, so they arrived earlier.

When he eventually had to continue on his journey after visiting her, he continued to write every day, in some cases so much that he had to use more than one pigeon. His beloved, however, was in despair. She noted that the pigeons were arriving later every day. She interpreted this as him forgetting about her. She thought he was instead thinking of the deals he would make in the next city or dealing with problems with the camels or something like that. She thought he then realized that he had forgotten to write, felt guilty, and wrote even more to try to make it up. In fact, the reason was much simpler: the pigeons had a longer distance to travel each day. If she had only understood that the Doppler effect affects pigeons just like it does sound waves, she would have had no reason for despair.

I have used this story for many years to explain the Doppler effect and have one amusing anecdote to relate. One year I was teaching three different courses simultaneously and was scheduled to discuss the Doppler effect in medical ultrasound in each of the courses. One afternoon I came to the least formal of the courses, which was a seminar on medical imaging techniques for graduate students in engineering. I had forgotten whether I had spoken to them about the Doppler effect, so I asked what I had already covered. There was silence. I asked if I had spoken about the Doppler effect. There was still silence. I asked if they had heard the story about the two sweethearts in the Middle East. They all started to nod and say yes! This just shows that even graduate students in engineering are more interested in love stories than in the Doppler effect!

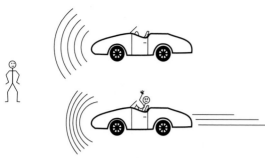

Figure 1–4. For the stationary sports car on the top, the distance between the pressure waves is determined by the frequency of the horn and the speed of sound. For the speeding sports car on the bottom, the distance between the pressure waves is shorter in the direction of travel because the car has moved by the time the horn creates the next pressure wave. The observer on the left will hear a higher frequency from the horn in the car moving towards him than from the horn in the stationary car.

All of us have experienced the change in pitch of an ambulance siren as it passes us or the change in pitch of the sound of a car or train passing us. As the vehicle is coming closer, the pitch is slightly higher, and when it is going away from us, the pitch of the sound is lower. There is a precise mathematic relationship between the velocity, speed of sound, and change in pitch. This can be understood if we consider the case of a vehicle moving toward us, which is transmitting a pure tone at a single frequency, f_0 (Fig. 1–4).

The tone being emitted consists of a sequence of pressure waves, with a period of $1/f_0$. The distance between the peaks of these waves is the wavelength. If the vehicle is stationary, the wavelength would be dependent on the velocity of sound c and would be c/f_0. By inverting the same process, we can demonstrate that the frequency with which these wave fronts will arrive at our ears will be f_0.

If the vehicle is moving toward us with a velocity of v, however, the distance between the waves will be $c/f_0 - v/f_0$, or the distance traveled by the sound in the period between waves minus the distance traveled by the vehicle. To determine the resulting frequency, f, we can use the fact that the resulting wavelength would be c/f, so:

$$c/f = c/f_0 - v/f_0$$
$$\text{or}$$
$$c/f = (c - v)/f_0$$

Thus,

$$f = f_0 c/(c - v)$$

The equation is often rewritten to express the difference between f and f_0, or Δf. So:

$$\Delta f = f - f_0 = f_0 c/(c - v) - f_0$$

Combining the terms on the right and eliminating those that cancel, yields:

$$\Delta f = v f_0/(c - v)$$

Because the speed of sound in blood is approximately 1560 m/s, and the highest velocities of interest in the heart are well under 10 m/s, the v in the denominator is not of major significance, and the equation is usually simplified by dropping the v in the denominator, for $\Delta f = f_0 v/c$. Another way of understanding this is that the change in frequency is equal to the fundamental frequency times the ratio between the velocity and the speed of sound.

An important point to recall is that only the component of the velocity in the direction of the receiver is of importance. If the actual direction of motion is not toward or away from the receiver, the actual change in frequency will be less, by a factor determined by the cosine of the angle (Fig. 1–5). This yields the equation:

$$\Delta f = \cos\theta f_0 v/c$$

We then have the equation that we will apply to measuring blood flow velocity, with one exception. The blood itself does not emit

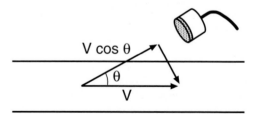

Figure 1–5. If the transducer beam is not pointed in the same direction as the flow of blood, the measured velocity will be less than the actual velocity. This is because the measured velocity is only the vector component of the true velocity (V) that is in the direction of the beam (Vcosθ).

sound but instead reflects sound that is transmitted toward it by the transducer. The Doppler effect will operate on the sound twice: once when it is "received" by the red cells before being reflected and again when it is reflected. This will result in a factor of two in the equation, so that the final equation will be

$$\Delta f = 2\cos\theta f_0 v/c$$

There are two important points to note about this equation. First, the measured velocity will be reduced if there is a significant angle between the direction of blood flow and the beam of ultrasound. The amount of this reduction will be small for small angles but becomes rapidly larger at larger angles (Fig. 1–6). It might seem very tempting to estimate the angle and correct for this reduction of the estimated velocity. Most ultrasound machines have software that allows the user to do this quite easily. This temptation should be resisted, however. The angle can only be estimated and that estimate has an error associated with it. The error introduced by this uncertainty of the angle estimate increases rapidly just as the potential benefit from angle correction becomes real. The conclusion is that angle correction is reliable when you do not need it and unreliable when you do need it! Instead, the operator should measure velocities from

several windows to obtain several estimates. The highest of these values should be used rather than using a good signal taken at a bad angle.

Second, the measured Doppler shift is directly proportional to the transmitted frequency. If the technique we are using is a pulsed technique (described later), the highest velocities we can measure will be reduced as the frequency of the transducer increases.

It may seem rather surprising that there is any backscattered signal from blood, because it appears dark in most imaging and the individual red cells are so much smaller than the wavelength of ultrasound used. In fact, the backscattered signal from blood is markedly weaker than that from tissue, and the backscatter can be accounted for by random variations in the number of red cells rather than the individual red cells themselves.

Measurement of Pressure Gradients

One of the most valuable uses for Doppler echocardiography is for the measurement of pressure gradients within the heart. Although this seems unlikely at first, this is based on something we have all experienced.

The principle is easily understood with a garden hose as an example. If there is no

Figure 1–6. Correcting for the angle of the Doppler beam relative to the flow would be fine if one knew the exact angle. Errors in the estimate of the angle are multiplicative and significant. The filled circles represent the error caused by the angle, if not corrected. The filled squares represent the error caused by correcting for angle, if there is a 10-degree inaccuracy in the angle estimate. For small angles the error resulting from correcting is actually greater than the error from not correcting, but even at large angles the error from correcting remains large.

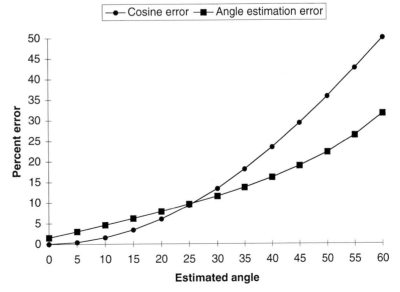

nozzle on the hose and we turn the water on, there will be a free flow of water but at a low velocity. If we put our thumb over the end of the hose, we can create a jet of higher velocity, and we can even control the velocity by the amount of pressure we exert. There is a relationship between the velocity of the jet and the pressure we exert, which we understand intuitively.

This relationship has a mathematic expression in the Bernoulli equation. The full equation actually has three terms, referred to as the viscous friction, flow acceleration, and convective acceleration terms. Only the last of these dominates for the situation of a small leak in a membrane (Fig. 1–7), which closely approximates both valvular stenosis and insufficiency. If we express the equation with only the convection acceleration term we have:

$$\Delta P = P_1 - P_2 = \rho(V_2^2 - V_1^2)/2$$

Where ΔP is the difference in pressure, ρ is the specific gravity of blood, and V_2 and V_1 are the velocity in the stenosis and proximal to the stenosis, respectively. If we measure the pressure gradient in millimeters of mercury, and the velocity of blood flow in meters per second, the equation can be expressed as:

$$\Delta P = 4(V_2^2 - V_1^2)$$

Finally, because the proximal velocity is often very low and close to 1, we can neglect it without major error in those situations, leading to the simplest form of the equation:

$$\Delta P = 4V_2^2$$

In this form, we can often calculate the pressure gradients in our head, especially if

Table 1–1. Anchor Values for Pressure Gradients

Velocity (m/s)	Pressure Gradient (mm Hg)
2.0	16
2.5	25
3.0	36
3.5	50
4.0	64
4.5	81
5.0	100

we use several easily remembered points as "anchors." These are listed in Table 1–1. Intermediate values can be readily estimated during the examination as a guide.

We will now review what kind of errors we can make with this technique (Box 1–4). Errors can be divided into underestimation of pressure gradients and overestimation of gradients. Underestimation is the easiest because there are two possibilities that are quite obvious and only one that is less obvious. The first is when the ultrasound beam is at a significant angle to the direction of blood flow, as is evident from the Doppler equation. The other is when we are not measuring in the center of the high velocity flow but just at the edges, where the flow velocity is lower. A third, less obvious cause of underestimation is when we have a long area of stenosis, such as in very small muscular ventricular septal defect. In these situations, the viscous term of the Bernoulli equation becomes much more significant in determining the gradient, but we have left it out of our simplified calculations.

Overestimation of gradients are slightly more complex, but there are also only three

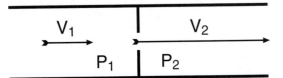

Figure 1–7. We understand that if there is a restrictive hole with a fluid flowing through it, there will be a difference in pressures. There will also be a difference in velocities, and there is a mathematical relationship between the two. See text for details.

BOX 1–4
POTENTIAL ERRORS IN ESTIMATING GRADIENTS

Underestimation resulting from

   Large angle between beam and flow

   Not measuring highest velocity

   Long, tubular channel

Overestimation resulting from

   High proximal velocity not measured

   Funnel-shaped obstruction

   Transit time effect

possible causes, again with two that are fairly clear and one that requires more explanation. The two related situations that are clear are based on elevation of the proximal velocity. In some situations, such as a coarctation of the aorta, the proximal velocity is significant, and ignoring it would lead to serious errors. Similar errors can occur if there is a narrow left ventricular outflow tract and mild aortic stenosis. This can also occur if there is a funnel shape leading to the opening. This will lead to a gradual acceleration, which results in less pressure gradient for a given velocity. This can occur in some congenital defects and with prosthetic valves.

The more complex issue is the transit time effect. This is an uncertainty in the estimation of very high velocities, which can lead to overestimation. Although the actual effect is rather complex, a simple analogy can help explain it (Fig. 1–8). If we were to measure the speed of a car using a stopwatch and timing when the car passed marks placed 100 yards apart on the pavement, we could obtain a fairly accurate estimate of the actual speed, subject to the errors occurring when we pressed the stopwatch button. We could express the speed and then calculate the estimated range of error based on the error in time of pressing the stopwatch button. For example, if we know that our time of pressing the button varied by up to 0.1 second in either direction and the time we recorded was 4.0 seconds, we could calculate the estimated velocity as 100 yards in the range of 3.9 to 4.1 seconds, or 24 to 26 yards per second, or 50 to 52

miles per hour. If, however, we were to reduce the distance to 10 yards, the error in time of pressing the stopwatch button would be much greater in proportion to the total measurement time, and our spread of values would be much larger. The time would be 0.4 seconds ±0.1 second, or 0.3 to 0.5 seconds. This would yield estimated speeds of 20 to 33 yards per second, or 41 to 68 miles per hour. Our estimated speed for the car would extend to a much higher value than in the first case.

In the situation of measuring blood flow with Doppler ultrasound, we are observing the velocity of groups of red blood cells. At high velocities, these cells may move through the sample volume for such a short time that we are unable to observe them for the full time required, and this leads to an uncertainty of the velocity, just as in the case with the car. The range of possible velocities is what will actually be displayed on the screen, and if we are identifying the peak velocity only for our measurements, we may overestimate the true velocity.

A number of other situations exist in which both catheter-derived gradients and Doppler gradients are correct but do not agree. The classic example of this is "peak-to-peak" gradients in aortic stenosis and maximum instantaneous gradients. The peak-to-peak gradient is frequently used as an easily estimated measure of stenosis severity. It is defined as the difference between the peak left ventricular pressure and the peak aortic pressure regardless of when these peaks occur. Unfortunately, the peak of aortic pressure is typically delayed in aortic stenosis; the time becomes later and later as the severity increases. This means that the peak-to-peak gradient is comparing pressures at different times in the cardiac cycle. The Doppler estimate is actually closer to reflecting the instantaneous gradient and may result in a much higher value. The solution is to compare mean gradients with the two techniques, which correlate very well.

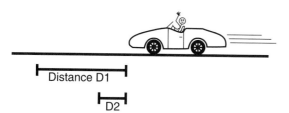

Figure 1–8. The transit time effect can be understood as the error in estimating velocity. If we time a car as it passes two marks (distance D1), the uncertainty in our measurement will be due to the variability in our pressing the button on the stopwatch. That uncertainty will be proportionally larger if the observation time is shorter because of the marks being closer together (D2).

Measurement of Flow

It is easier to understand the connection between flow velocity and total flow than the connection between pressure gradients and velocity. If we imagine a circular bar moving longitudinally past us, it is easy to see that the volume of bar per unit time will be equal to the cross-section of the bar times the velocity (distance per unit time). If we substitute a fluid flowing in a pipe, with a uniform velocity across the cross-section, the same relationship will be true. The volume flow rate will be equal to the velocity times the cross-sectional area. What is equally true, but not as obvious, is that this relationship is true for any distribution of velocity and area as long as we match up areas with the flow in the area; that is, the integral over the cross-section of velocity times time results in volumetric flow.

To apply this to the clinical situation, the assumption is usually made that the velocity of blood flow is uniform across the cross-section of interest. This is based on the theory in hydrodynamics that the profile will be flat in regions of acceleration. If this is true, we can multiply the velocity measured at one point multiplied by the cross-sectional area to obtain the volumetric flow (Fig. 1–9). For example, we can measure the velocity of flow in the aortic annulus and the diameter of the aortic annulus. Assuming the annulus is round, we can calculate the cross-sectional area. Assuming that the velocity is uniform, the area times the velocity will equal volumetric flow.

Of course, flow in the heart is more complex than that. A major difference is that it is pulsatile, with periods of no flow and periods of high flow. We can calculate the mean flow by integrating the velocity over time and dividing by time. We can then multiply this mean velocity times the cross-sectional area we have calculated to derive the flow rate.

A more convenient way of doing this is to calculate the velocity integral over time (the velocity-time integral, or VTI, also called the time-velocity integral, or TVI). If we multiply this times the cross-sectional area, we obtain the stroke volume, and then by multiplying with the heart rate, we obtain the cardiac output.

Unfortunately, the cross-sectional velocity profiles in the heart are usually not flat. This can lead to significant errors in the estimation of the volumetric flow rate. Newer techniques may result in a more accurate estimate of volumetric flow, based on the quantitative data inherent in color Doppler.

Another use of the volumetric flow is the estimation of stenotic valve areas using the continuity equation (see Fig. 1–9). This calculation is based on conservation of volume. If we can estimate the total flow in a channel, such as the left ventricular outflow tract, and all of that flow is going through a stenotic orifice, the total flow through the orifice must be the same. If we measure the velocity in the orifice, we should be able to back calculate the area of the orifice:

$$A_1V_1 = \text{flow} = A_2V_2$$
$$A_2 = A_1V_1/V_2$$

Because there are errors in all of the measurements, as noted previously, the total error can be significant; nevertheless, this calculation can give an objective estimate of the severity of a stenosis, especially if there is a low output state.

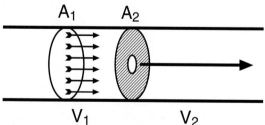

Figure 1–9. We can estimate the flow in a channel by measuring the cross-sectional area and flow velocity. By assuming a uniform velocity of flow across the cross-section, we can calculate the flow as velocity times area: $V_1 \times A_1$. If there is a narrowing downstream, we can also estimate the area by measuring the velocity through the narrowing: $A_2 = (V_1 \times A_1)/V_2$. See text for details.

Continuous Wave

In practice, there are two fundamentally different ways of producing and measuring a Doppler shift, called continuous-wave and pulsed-wave Doppler. The simplest, conceptually, is continuous-wave Doppler. In this method, two transducers are used. One transmits a continuous signal, hence the name. The other transducer is directed so that its range of sensitivity overlaps with the first and receives continuously (Fig. 1–10). This received signal is used to measure the Doppler shift from the transmitted signal.

The signal is usually analyzed in short sequences of time, commonly 5 ms. The calculated velocity is displayed on the Y axis, whereas the strength of the signal is displayed as the brightness of the display. Successive 5-ms intervals are displayed along the horizontal axis to create a so-called spectral Doppler display (Fig. 1–11), because it is based on the frequency spectrum of the returning ultrasound signal.

Continuous-wave Doppler is capable of measuring the highest velocities we can measure in the heart and can be quite easy to use because we only need to point the transducer in the direction we wish to measure and do not need to choose a depth. This strength is also its major weakness, because we are unable to select a depth and, therefore, do no know from which depth the signal is coming. In most cases, however, either there is only one possible source or changing the angle of the transducer or other cues makes only one source possible.

An example of only one possible source is if we measure a holosystolic high velocity

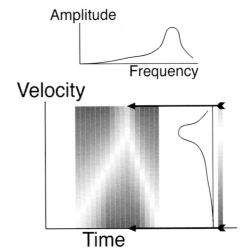

Figure 1–11. Each vertical column of the spectral display represents the spectrum of frequencies at a given time period; the amplitude is represented as brightness on the display. The upper curve represents a spectral curve from one point in time, with the frequency on the horizontal axis and the amplitude on the vertical axis. We can image this curve rotated so that the frequency is in the vertical direction, on the lower right. If the amplitude is then converted to brightness, we have one vertical line of the spectral display. A sequence of such vertical components constitutes the spectral display (lower left).

directed toward the transducer in the parasternal position; this would be ventricular septal defect. If we measure a high velocity from the right parasternal or suprasternal notch, this could either be due to aortic ste-

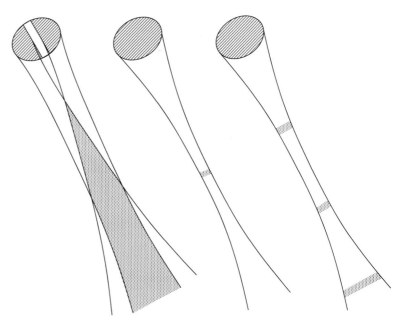

Figure 1–10. Continuous-wave Doppler is measured using two transducers: one for transmitting and one for receiving (left). Their beams overlap over a large area, so there is uncertainty about the source of the Doppler signal. Low-pulse-repetition-rate Doppler has very high spatial resolution but at the cost of not being able to measure high velocities (center). High-pulse-repetition-rate Doppler has some spatial ambiguity because of multiple sample volumes but is able to measure higher velocities (right).

nosis or mitral regurgitation. We could distinguish between these two by noting the duration of the signal. Aortic stenosis would be much shorter than mitral regurgitation because the mitral regurgitation would continue in the isovolumetric contraction and relaxation phases of the cardiac cycle.

Pulsed Wave

Pulsed-wave Doppler can be performed with a single transducer, much like imaging (see Fig. 1–10). A pulse of ultrasound energy is transmitted (hence the name), and then the same transducer is used to receive the returning signal. By "listening" to the returning ultrasound signal at a specified time after the instrument sent the pulse, it is possible to limit the analysis to a specific depth. This limiting process is called "gating" of the Doppler signal. However, one such transmitted and received pulse is not

sufficient to analyze the Doppler shift, so a sequence of pulses is sent out. The rate at which these pulses are sent out is called the pulse repetition frequency (PRF).

In many ways, this process is similar to observing motion with a stroboscopic light. Each pulse of ultrasonic energy corresponds to a flash of the strobe light. If an object is moving or oscillating slowly, we can accurately perceive its motion. If it is moving rapidly, however, we may perceive it as moving in a different direction or in a jerky fashion. This phenomenon is called aliasing and can be understood through a simple analogy. Most of us have seen a western film in which there is a stagecoach or wagon, and the wheels appeared to be rotating backward. This too is aliasing and can help us understand the phenomenon. It occurs because the camera is also only observing intermittently, like our ultrasound pulses. If the degree of motion between frames of film is small, our brain is able

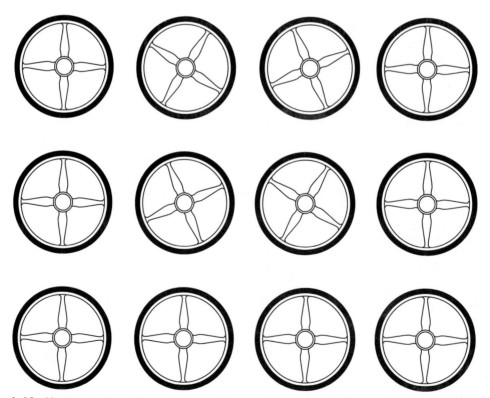

Figure 1–12. Aliasing can be understood using, as an example, wagon wheels in a western film. If the rate of rotation is slow enough, our brains can connect the individual frames and deduce the clockwise rotation in the top row by one-twelfth turn in each of the frames, until we have one-quarter turn on the right. If the rotation is too fast (one-sixth rotation per frame in the middle row), it looks as if the rotation is reversed (middle row). At some rotational rates, such as one-quarter rotation per frame in the bottom row, the wheel appears to be standing still.

to make the correct assumption about the direction of motion (Fig. 1–12). If the rate of rotation is higher, it can make the wheel appear to stand still or even rotate in the wrong direction. Above a certain rotational rate, the perception will not be accurate. If we had been looking at the wagon or stagecoach in person, however, the wheels would have always appeared to rotate in the correct direction because our eyes effectively observe continuously. In much the same way, continuous-wave Doppler correctly identifies high velocities, whereas with pulsed-wave Doppler the velocities will appear incorrectly on the display or even in the opposite direction if the velocity exceeds a certain value (Fig. 1–13).

The speed at which this misperception of the motion, or aliasing, occurs is dependent on the rate of transmitted pulses, or PRF. This is adjusted so that each transmitted pulse is able to return after traveling the depth to the area of interest. The returning signal is gated, as noted previously, so that only signals from a given depth are ana-

lyzed. This means that if we are examining a deep structure, the transmission time for the ultrasound will be longer, and the PRF will, therefore, be lower, and aliasing will occur at a lower frequency. The frequency at which aliasing occurs is often called the Nyquist limit. This limit is at a frequency equal to one-half of the PRF.

This aliasing *frequency* is related to the aliasing *velocity* by the Doppler equation. We can take this further by using the formulas we derived before and defining the depth of interest as d. The travel time of a single pulse to depth d would be 2d/c. The PRF would be the inverse of this, or c/2d, and the maximum frequency we could measure without aliasing would be half that, or c/4d. If we substitute this into the Doppler equation as the change in frequency and rearranging the terms, we can then calculate the maximum velocity that can be measured by pulsed Doppler without aliasing, as a function of the depth, frequency, and speed of sound.

$$c/4d = 2vf_0/c$$
$$v = c^2/8f_0d$$

We could send out another pulse before the first has returned. This technique is called high PRF (HPRF) Doppler, and the first technique described is termed low PRF (LPRF) Doppler to distinguish it. If we send out pulses at twice the LPRF rate, we can measure velocities up to twice the LPRF velocity limit. We will also measure velocities that originate at a location one-half the distance to our original region of interest, and these signals will be indistinguishable from those coming from our true region of interest. The process can be continued further, so that we send out pulses at three times the LPRF rate, but then we have two additional sample volumes at shorter distances. In general, we lose spatial specificity as we gain high-velocity specificity.

Both LPRF and HPRF Doppler can define the location of the flow being measured, but HPRF Doppler is capable of measuring higher velocities, approaching those measured by continuous wave. These techniques can be more difficult to use in practice because the operator must not only have the

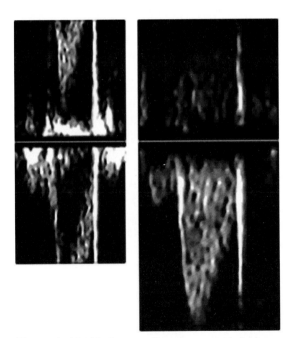

Figure 1–13. Aliasing can affect the spectral display as well. This example shows aortic valve flow measured from the apex. A pulsed system *(left)* will have a velocity limit and will display velocities over that limit in the reverse direction as coming toward the transducer, whereas a continuous-wave Doppler system *(right)* will display the velocities correctly.

transducer beam pointed in the correct direction but must also have the sample volume set at the correct depth. When looking for a specific signal, there are three dimensions to search in, rather than just two, and, therefore, that much more of a chance to miss a signal of interest (Box 1–5).

Color Flow Mapping

The technique commonly called color flow mapping, or color Doppler flow mapping, is actually a two-dimensional Doppler velocity estimation technique, but the results are usually presented in colors on the screen. So even though two-dimensional Doppler velocity mapping would be a more informative name, we will use the term color Doppler flow mapping or color flow mapping because these are the most common usages.

In the preceding section on pulsed-wave Doppler, the concept of gating was introduced. A pulse of ultrasound is transmitted in a given direction, and although echoes are received continuously from different depths, we choose to listen at only a specified time, "gating" the signal so that only that part is analyzed. In a very simplified view of what is done in color Doppler imaging, we need add only two elements to this model. The first is multiple gating, in which we listen at multiple depths simultaneously to create a spectrum for each depth. The second is to sweep the beam through the sector so we can have spectral data for the entire sector.

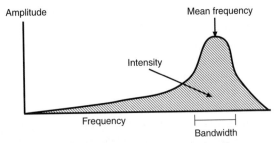

Figure 1–14. Color flow mapping is only able to extract limited information about each pixel. The spectrum is summarized as the intensity of the Doppler signal (area under the curve), the mean frequency, and the width of the distribution (bandwidth).

In broad strokes, this is exactly what is done for color flow mapping. In detail, many compromises must be made. In the previous section on pulsed-wave Doppler, it was pointed out that as many as 128 pulses may be sent in a given direction and that the time for this to be done is dependent on the time of transmission for the ultrasound through tissue. If we use a depth of 10 cm, each pulse must travel 20 cm. If the instrument is transmitting 128 pulses in each direction and 128 beams are used to generate one image, the total time to collect one color image would be $128 \times 128 \times 20$ cm/1560 m/s or 2.1 seconds. Clearly, we must transmit fewer pulses.

If we send very few pulses in each direction, we cannot calculate a full spectrum and must instead be satisfied with a more limited estimate of the spectral values. This usually consists of an estimate of the mean velocity, bandwidth, and amplitude (Fig. 1–14). The mean velocity is normally the average velocity in the sample volume being represented, but if the bandwidth is high, this cannot be accurately estimated, and the value returned is actually random. The bandwidth is an estimate of the dispersion of velocities within the sample volume. There may be turbulence or shear forces that cause different flow rates in different parts of the sample volume. In addition, aliasing, if present, can also show up as an increased bandwidth. Finally, there is the strength of the signal, which is primarily dependent on the strength of the ultrasound transmission to the given depth but can also be diminished at very low flow rates owing

---

BOX 1–5
TYPES OF DOPPLER

Continuous-wave
  Very high velocities can be measured
  Low spatial resolution
Low pulse repetition frequency (including color flow mapping)
  Aliasing of high velocities
  High spatial resolution
High pulse repetition frequency
  High velocities can be measured
  Some spatial ambiguity

to the low-velocity filter (also called low-velocity reject, high-pass filter, or wall filter). This is used to limit the very strong signals from slow-moving structures in the heart.

Fortunately, this limitation of values helps us with another problem: how to simultaneously display a large number of spectral Doppler signals. Because there are only the three values mentioned previously, we can combine them into a color for each pixel, even though the data used to create the colors are actually quantitative velocity information.

Because our information is so limited, we cannot interpret distributions of flow velocities as accurately as in the case with spectral Doppler. Also, because the technique is a pulsed technique, with a low pulse repetition rate, it will be subject to aliasing at low velocities. Both aliasing and turbulent flow will cause a wide bandwidth, and in both of these circumstances the mean velocity estimate will be a random number. Because of this, it is probably best to term this type of flow "disturbed," because we cannot extract much more information from it. The appearance of such flow will depend on the instrument. On some, the random nature of the velocity estimate leads to random colors, which has been called a "mosaic" or "confetti" pattern. Other instruments add green or yellow when there is high bandwidth, so that the appearance may be one of these colors. Many instruments even allow the user to change the settings of how the velocity and bandwidth are combined to create the colors. Smooth flow of low velocity will result in a low bandwidth and an accurate mean velocity estimate and direction and, therefore, more uniform colors.

Color flow mapping is particularly helpful for demonstrating relationships of flow, identifying disturbed flow, and screening large areas quickly (Box 1–6). An example of demonstrating relationships of flow is showing that there is continuity of flow across the atrial septum from the left to the right atrium, which is strongly supportive evidence for the diagnosis of atrial septal defect. Evidence of disturbed flow, with a high bandwidth, may be the first indication we have for a small muscular ventricular

---

BOX 1–6
ADVANTAGES OF COLOR FLOW MAPPING
Demonstrates spatial relationships of flow
Identifies disturbed flow
Screens large areas

---

septal defect that would otherwise be missed.

Color Doppler has significant drawbacks that can result in misunderstanding of flow relations or even misdiagnosis. These have to do with the low frame rate of color Doppler imaging and the large amount of information presented to the observer, as well as the many variables that can affect the sensitivity of the color Doppler imaging. These can lead to missing an abnormality because of the low frame rate and high degree of information or false-positive results caused by high gain or weak signal.

Pitfalls and Artifacts

We have already examined some of the sources of error that can affect each of the individual techniques. Some pitfalls can affect all ultrasound techniques, although in slightly different ways. These must also be understood to avoid serious errors of interpretation.

Side Lobe Artifacts

Perhaps the most important and least understood artifact is caused by the side lobes of the ultrasound beam. It is easy to consider the image we see on the ultrasound screen as a "slice" through the anatomic structures; however, the cross-section that is generated is much more complex than that.

The beam of ultrasound that is generated is often considered to have a finite width, which is a function of the transducer frequency, diameter, and shape. As a general rule, the width is narrower with higher frequencies and larger diameter of the trans-

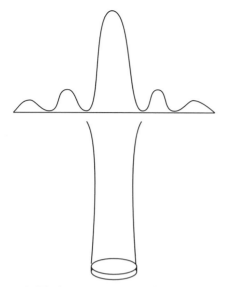

Figure 1–15. Side lobes are areas of sensitivity that point in directions other than the main beam direction. Even though the transducer is pointed straight up, and we imagine the beam as being pointed that way as well (below), there are areas of sensitivity to the sides in all directions, illustrated in the sensitivity plot above. If a very echogenic structure falls in one of these areas, an image will be generated but in the direction the beam is pointing, not the true location.

ducer. The echoes received by the ultrasound instrument are a sum of the echoes generated within this finite width slice. This width, however, refers only to the width of the main lobe of the intensity distribution, as shown in Figures 1–1 and 1–15. A number of weaker side lobes can also contribute. It is easiest to understand what consequences this will have in two-dimensional imaging.

For most echo targets, the intensity of the echo from the main lobe is moderate. Because the intensity of the echo from the side lobes is much less, we will most probably be unable to detect it. If there is a very strong echo reflector, the echo from the side lobes will be measurable and will result in an image as well. If the strong scatterer is in the plane of the image, it will result in a blurring of the image in a circumferential direction. This is because the echoes will return even when the beam is pointed slightly to the side, and the instrument will display the echo as if it had come from the main lobe direction (i.e., to the side). This spreading of the image is usually easy to

detect because there is always the bright echo in the center, with blurring on either side.

The situation is different if the bright reflector is outside of the plane of imaging. Side lobes occur in all directions, even out of the plane of imaging. In that situation, it may not be possible to see the bright echo coming from the strong scatterer but only the weaker side lobe echoes. These may be mistaken for an actual structure, with confusing, or even serious consequences.

The primary method of identifying confusing echoes as coming from side lobe artifacts in any echo technique is to direct the scan plane in adjacent positions, looking for the bright source of the artifact. If none can be identified, it is virtually impossible for the echoes to be due to a side lobe. Similarly, if the suspect echo is still visible in the same location from a very different echo window, it is very unlikely to be a side lobe artifact.

Another method that is also useful for distinguishing side lobe artifacts in two-dimensional imaging is to change the transducer frequency. Because the size and position of side lobes is determined by the relationship between the frequency and the size of the transducer, changing these should change the appearance of any side lobe artifact dramatically or even cause it to disappear. If the confusing echo is caused by an actual structure, the appearance will be changed only slightly, as is to be expected with changes in transducer frequency (Box 1–7).

Side lobe artifacts can affect Doppler

BOX 1–7
IDENTIFICATION OF SIDE LOBE ARTIFACTS

Scan adjacent planes

    Echogenic source of side lobe artifact can be identified

Scan other windows

    Artifact not found in same location

Change transducer frequency

    Artifact moves, gets worse with lower frequency or better with higher frequency

measurements as well. In the case of Doppler, we could measure a flow that is not in the anatomic plane we are imaging. Examples of this include measuring superior vena cava flow from the subcostal position while imaging the interatrial septum. The appearance is that of flow across the septum, suggesting an interatrial septal defect or fenestrated septum. As is the case when imaging side lobe artifacts, the key to correct identification is to search for the image source, in this case the superior vena cava. By angling the imaging plane, we can see whether the superior vena cava flow is just adjacent to and identical with the flow we suspect to be across the atrial septum. If not, the flow cannot be explained as a side lobe artifact. As mentioned in Chapter 5, physiological details can also be used to distinguish superior vena cava from atrial septal defect flow.

Reflection Artifacts

Some structures act almost like mirrors, reflecting the ultrasound energy very efficiently and preserving the relationships of the ultrasound wave fronts. This can result in mirror-like images of structures. The classic example of this phenomenon is the appearance of a ventricle-like structure posterior to the heart in the parasternal view, caused by multiple reflection from the pericardium (Fig. 1–16). The image is in fact of the left ventricle, and the motions are identical. In addition, the distances from the reflecting structure to the reflected image are identical to the distance of the structure from the reflecting surface as well. This leads us to the characteristics that can identify a reflection artifact. A strong echo reflector must be visible. The motions of the suspect echo are congruent with the visible structures and are present at a multiple of the distance from the echogenic structure. Finally, the suspect structure is not seen, or not seen in the same place, when imaging is performed from a completely different window (Box 1–8).

The same sort of effect can be seen with Doppler as well as imaging. An example of this is the appearance of a second "channel" posterior to the true aorta when viewed

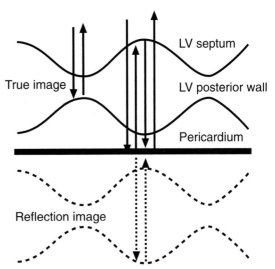

Figure 1–16. Reflection artifacts result from multiple reflection of ultrasound from very efficient reflectors, such as pericardium. Because the reflected ultrasound takes a longer path, the instrument indicates an echo at a larger depth. This schematic illustrates the situation for M-mode of the left ventricle (LV) if the pericardium is very echogenic. At the upper left, true reflections from the myocardium are illustrated. In the middle, an incoming pulse, which is reflected from the pericardium, is shown. It is then reflected by the left ventricular septum back toward the pericardium and then reflected by the pericardium back to the transducer. Because of the long time of flight for this pulse when it is received again by the transducer, it is displayed at a greater depth, shown below, creating a reflection image.

from the suprasternal notch (Fig. 1–17; see also color figure). The structural image shows an echolucent area, suggesting a vascular structure. The color Doppler also shows flow, consistent with arterial flow. Even pulsed Doppler placed in the artifact will show normal arterial flow patterns. This is a reflection artifact caused by the total internal reflection of the ultrasound

---

BOX 1–8
IDENTIFYING REFLECTION ARTIFACTS

Source of reflection is visible

Found at same distance from reflector as real structure

Congruent motion with real structure and reflector

Not found from other windows

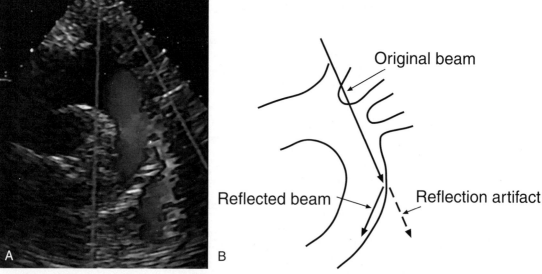

Figure 1–17. Reflection can also affect Doppler signals. *A* (also see color figure), In a suprasternal view of the aortic arch, it is possible to see the color flow in the descending aorta. There also appears to be color flow exiting from the aorta and even visible in a "channel" located posterior to the aorta. *B,* Diagram explaining this observation. The posterior wall of the aorta causes the ultrasound beam to be reflected toward the descending aorta. This reflection affects both the tissue image, resulting in the "channel" and the color Doppler flow. Sampling with pulsed-wave Doppler in this "channel" would demonstrate normal descending aortic flow.

beam by the inside of the aortic wall. All of the ultrasound signals caused are consistent with the "reality" of the signal because they are caused by the real descending aorta, seen in a reflection. The key to identifying this artifact is recognition that it can occur and identification of the structure causing the reflection.

This type of artifact should be considered whenever there is an unexpected "extra" structure seen.

Reverberation Artifacts

Reverberation artifacts are perhaps the easiest to identify. They are caused by very dense echogenic structures, which cause a very large number of multiple reflections. Thus, in a sense, they are related to reflection artifacts. The difference is that the number of repeated reflections is so large that there is no clear image formed. What appears instead is a "clutter" of echoes, which can appear like some space-filling structure. This type of artifact is usually caused by calcifications or some prosthetic material (Fig. 1–18). Reverberation will also

disturb the Doppler signal but not in a simple, predictable way.

ECHOCARDIOGRAPHIC VIEWS AND METHOD OF EXAMINATION

The flexibility of the transthoracic echocardiographic examination can lead to confusion because there are many different positions in which to place the transducer and a virtually infinite number of variations in the orientation of the transducer in each location. In addition, it is necessary to be able to communicate with others how the view was obtained. For this reason, there are a number of standard views and a standard way of naming and displaying those views. Views are named based on the location of the transducer on the patient and the orientation of the plane of imaging relative to the heart. The locations where the transducers are placed are those that allow transmission of ultrasound without intervening lung or bone. The most common locations used are the left parasternal, subcostal, apical, and suprasternal "windows"

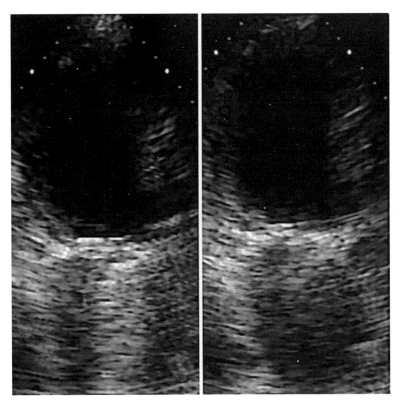

Figure 1–18. Reverberation is a form of multiple reflection caused by strongly echogenic materials, usually artificial. In the left image, a mechanical prosthetic mitral valve causes intense reverberation echoes almost filling the left atrium during systole in the apical two-chamber view. This could possibly be mistaken for a left atrial mass. On the right is the same view during diastole, when the valve is open. The revereberation echoes are markedly diminished because the leaflets of the prosthesis are in the open position and more parallel to the ultrasound beam.

(Fig. 1–19). Less common, but sometimes useful, windows include the right parasternal, supraclavicular, infraclavicular, and, for dextrocardia, the right apical windows.

The orientation of the scanning plane relative to the heart is based on the orientation of the ventricles of the heart. If we view the left ventricle as a type of cylinder, we can imagine that it has a length and cross-section

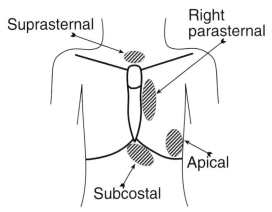

Figure 1–19. The most common echocardiographic windows are the suprasternal, right parasternal, subcostal, and apical windows.

tion (Fig. 1–20). If we view the plane that shows the cross-section of the cylinder, this is called the short-axis view. The long axis of the left ventricle as cylinder can have a number of different views, and three are commonly given names. All of these are obtainable from the apex. If the plane of view demonstrates the right ventricle and right atrium as well as the left ventricle and left atrium, the view is called the four-chamber view. If the view includes the left atrium and left ventricle only but also shows the aortic valve and ascending aorta, it is called the long-axis view. If only the left atrium and left ventricle are visible, it is called the two-chamber view. All of these views are aligned with the long axis of the left ventricle.

Not all views can be obtained from all windows, although virtually every view is obtainable from more than one window (Box 1–9). The complete name of a view is composed of the window and the view, such as parasternal long axis or apical four chamber. The final detail is the orientation of the images in the anteroposterior and left-right directions.

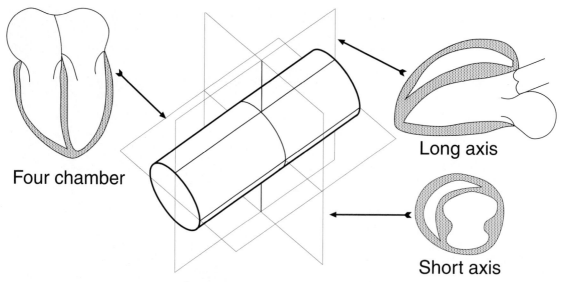

Four chamber

Long axis

Short axis

Figure 1–20. The orientation of echocardiographic views are named as if the left ventricle is a cylinder. The short-axis view is like a cross-section of the cylinder, and the views along the long axis are named the four chamber, long axis, and two chamber (not shown). See Appendix A for a more detailed presentation of echocardiographic views.

Echocardiography generally follows the conventions used in anatomy and radiology. The right side of the patient is displayed on the left of the screen, just as if we were looking at the patient directly or at a picture of the patient. Anterior and posterior views are displayed on the top and bottom of the image, respectively. The head direction (cephalad) is displayed on the top if we also see the right-left direction (just like looking at a picture) or to the right if the other direction is anteroposterior. The apical views are somewhat of an anomaly because the transducer is so far lateral. In these cases, the apex is often displayed on the top of the image, with the left-sided structures to the right of the image.

It should be noted that many other authors do not follow these conventions and may reverse right and left relative to what is described or display the apex down or even reverse the subcostal views. In addition, there is a question as to whether some of the oblique echocardiographic views from the apical and subcostal views are properly considered variants of anteroposterior views, with the head direction superior on the image, or are variants of cross-sectional images, with the anterior direction displayed superior on the image. These views are typically presented differently in pediatric and adult cardiology. In this book, when there is a difference between the prevalent presentation in pediatric and adult cardiology, both orientations are shown. See Appendix A for a more detailed presentation of the main echocardiographic views and variations of presentation.

The method of examination varies based on the age of the patient and is discussed in the following chapters, but some general comments are in order. Two different orien-

---

BOX 1–9
ECHOCARDIOGRAPHIC VIEWS

Parasternal
  Short axis
  Long axis
Apical
  Long axis
  Four chamber
  Two chamber
Subcostal
  Short axis
  Four chamber
Supraclavicular
  Aortic arch

tations of the operator and equipment relative to the patient are in common use. Some echocardiography laboratories prefer scanning with all of the equipment on the patient's left, using the left hand to hold the transducer and the operator facing the patient, whereas others prefer to scan with the equipment on the patient's right, using the right hand, again facing the patient. In my opinion, it makes little difference which way the scanning is done. However, there is an advantage to being able to do both in some situations when performing a portable examination, such as in the newborn intensive care unit, because one arrangement or the other may be more suited to the location of other equipment surrounding the patient, such as ventilators. In some particularly difficult situations, it may even be necessary to scan facing the patient's feet! In any case, there is an advantage in developing flexibility and learning to scan "ambidextrously."

THE INTEGRATED EXAMINATION REVISITED

Now that we have discussed the major techniques used in diagnostic cardiac ultrasound, we will see how they can fit together in a complementary way. Some of this requires an understanding of physiology as well, which is covered in more detail in Chapter 2. In even the most simple diagnoses, making the anatomic diagnosis is only half of the task to be accomplished in the echocardiographic examination. The other, and equally important, task is to determine the physiological consequences of the lesion. In some cases, knowledge of the expected physiology and finding a pattern that deviates from that can lead us to modify our diagnoses or find an unexpected additional defect.

If we have a patient with a suspected ventricular septal defect, we can use all of the modalities to make or confirm the diagnosis, but some will be more useful than others depending on the details of the patient's condition. Color Doppler is perhaps the technique that first comes to mind for the identification of a shunt lesion, and it is

in fact quite useful. In the case of a ventricular septal defect with high velocity flow, there will be aliasing that will be displayed as "disturbed flow" in a mosaic or green color. This will usually be quite apparent on the display. Because of the wide field of view, multiple ventricular septal defects can also be easily identified, even if the focus of attention is not directed at them. Finding such multiple defects can be difficult with the other techniques we would use.

Color Doppler has its weaknesses, however. Disturbed flow can have many causes, and small disturbances may be mistaken for small ventricular septal defects. The low frame rate can also make timing of events difficult. All of these problems combined with side lobe artifacts and reflection can lead to false-positive diagnoses. If there is an overreliance on color, one can also miss a large ventricular septal defect with equalization of pressures and "undisturbed" flow across it.

LPRF Doppler has the advantage of more clearly delineating the timing of events, because a new vertical line in the display is generated about 200 times each second. It is unable to unequivocally identify high-velocity flows because it is subject to aliasing. An additional problem with LPRF Doppler is that the operator must not only have the beam pointed in the right direction but also must have the sample volume at the correct depth. This additional adjustment increases the risk of missing the important flow that is being looked for.

Continuous-wave Doppler has the advantage of correctly identifying high velocities. This means that the direction of flow, the peak pressure difference, and pattern of pressure difference should be identifiable in most cases. In our example of a ventricular septal defect, if the defect is restrictive, we would expect a high velocity flow because of the high pressure difference between the right and left ventricles. The pattern of flow through a ventricular septal defect is quite characteristic and can help with making the diagnosis. We would still have the problem of a large defect with low-velocity flow, but we can partially compensate for this by looking for signs of higher pressures on the right side of the heart, such as a high-velocity tricuspid insufficiency jet. If we are able to find tricuspid insufficiency and the measured velocity is high, we know that there is a risk of missing a ventricular septal defect because the pressure difference between the ventricles is reduced. If, in contrast, we find tricuspid insufficiency and the velocity is low, and we do not find high velocity or disturbed flow in the vicinity of the ventricular septum, our negative finding carries much more weight.

HPRF Doppler is in many ways a blend of the characteristics of continuous-wave Doppler and LPRF Doppler. We have the advantages and disadvantages of localization of flow, with the advantages of measuring high-velocity flow.

Imaging has the advantage of showing large defects clearly but does not give us any information about the physiology. There is also a resolution limit to what we can find with imaging, which is probably on the order of 3 mm. This means, however, that it is sensitive in exactly the situations when Doppler may miss a ventricular septal defect (i.e., when the defect is large and there is equalization of the pressures).

In summary, for a ventricular septal defect: (1) color Doppler can easily identify multiple defects or defects with high-velocity flow as a result of high-pressure gradients, although there are problems with false-positive and false-negative results; (2) continuous-wave Doppler can clearly identify the physiology of restrictive defects and, therefore, has less of a problem with false-positive results but has more false-negative results; (3) LPRF Doppler has better time resolution than color Doppler and, therefore, can avoid some false-positive results but is unable to identify high-velocity flow patterns and requires adjustment of the depth as well as direction of the beam; (4) HPRF Doppler combines some of the advantages and disadvantages of continuous-wave and LPRF Doppler, with identification of high velocities, but the requirement of choosing the depth as well; (5) all Doppler techniques may miss large defects because there is no high-velocity or disturbed flow; (6) imaging can identify large lesions but can easily miss small ones.

The advantages and disadvantages of the different modalities are summarized in Table 1–2. Further examples of how the modalities are complementary are presented in the chapters that follow.

THE ECHOCARDIOGRAPHIC SURVEY EXAMINATION

One should attempt to confirm a number of findings on the echocardiographic exami-

Table 1–2. Characteristics of Different Techniques

Technique	Advantages	Disadvantages
M-mode imaging	Structure High time resolution	Difficult anatomic relations Little physiology
Sector imaging	Structure Anatomic relations	Low frame rate Little physiology
LPRF Doppler	Blood flow Localized measurement	Low limit on highest velocity Need to set depth as well as direction
HPRF Doppler	Blood flow Localized measurement High-velocity measurements Pressure gradients	Need to set depth as well as direction Some depth ambiguity
CW Doppler	Blood flow High-velocity measurements Pressure gradients	No localization of depth
Color Doppler	Blood flow relations Identification of unexpected	Low frame rate Low limit on highest velocity
Color M-mode	Blood flow relations No need to set depth High time resolution	Low limit on highest velocity

LPRF, low pulse repetition frequency; HPRF, high pulse repetition frequency; CW, continuous wave.

nation for each patient because these findings determine key points of the anatomy or physiology. Depending on the echocardiographic windows available, the particular view we use to confirm the findings may be different. This list of findings forms a sort of checklist, called the echocardiographic survey. The details of what is normal and what abnormalities we may find differ for the various age groups and are discussed in each chapter, but the basic principle is the same.

Most of the items have to do with confirming the presence and function of the major structures in the heart (Box 1–10). Identification of each of these structures and confirmation of normal function will rule out a large number of defects. Assessment of the right ventricular pressure is important for assessing not only the severity of many conditions but also the probability of missing some other types of defects.

Briefly, one should identify that there are two ventricles and an intact interventricular septum and examine the relative size of the two ventricles. Two atria should be identified and their relative size and the atrial septum assessed. Two atrioventricular valves should be present, each emptying into a different ventricle, and the tricuspid valve should be slightly closer to the apex than the mitral valve. Both should be opening well and not have significant insufficiency. The semilunar valves also are each associated with a ventricle and should be of relatively the same size and free of significant narrowing or leakage. The great arteries should cross, and the pulmonary artery should originate anteriorly, heading posteriorly. The aorta should originate posterior to the pulmonary artery and course cephalad toward the aortic arch. There should not be any significant flow acceleration in either

---

| **Box 1–10** |
| **THE ECHOCARDIOGRAPHIC** |
| **SURVEY EXAMINATION** |

Two ventricles
  Interventricular septum
  Relative size
Two atria
  Interatrial septum
  Relative size
Two atrioventricular valves
  Relative placement
  Stenosis/insufficiency
Two semilunar valves
  Connection to ventricles
  Stenosis/insufficiency
Great arteries
  Location
  Connections (ductus)
  Stenoses (coarctation/peripheral pulmonic stenosis)
Right ventricular pressure estimate
  Tricuspid insufficiency
  Pulmonic insufficiency

---

the aorta or the pulmonary branches. There should not be any retrograde flow in the pulmonary artery resulting from a ductus. Finally, the right ventricular peak systolic pressure should be estimated. If it is elevated, the risk of missing a shunt lesion is greater.

In most clinical situations, normal findings for each element of the survey examination will rule out significant disease. In all cases, the survey examination will provide the basis for a detailed diagnosis and evaluation.

Simplified Nomenclature and Physiology of Congenital Heart Disease

A major obstacle for the beginner learning about congenital heart disease is the confusing and sometimes inconsistent nomenclature. Combine this with unfamiliar concepts of the physiology of shunts, and the task may seem virtually unachievable, if not impossible.

Fortunately, the spectrum of actual cardiac defects is limited and amenable to organization. Certain defects appear together in constellations known as syndromes. Many of these syndromes can be further organized based on other principles to simplify the task further. Finally, the physiology can be broken down into simpler parts, which can be individually understood and then combined into a total understanding.

In this chapter, we first outline the fundamental, isolated congenital defects that can occur and the different names that can be applied to the same defects. We then learn some simple embryological mnemonics that can help us remember the details of most of the constellations of cardiac defects that occur together. We then discuss a simple way of looking at the physiology of cardiac defects to understand what we should be looking for in any lesion we might encounter.

ISOLATED ABNORMALITIES

Most of the congenital defects we encounter can be classified as a defect (hole), stenosis (narrowing causing obstruction), hypoplasia/atresia (underdevelopment or absence), or transposition/inversion/anomalous connection (wrong connection) (Box 2–1). We can further subdivide each of these

> **BOX 2-1**
> **CLASSIFICATION OF MOST ISOLATED ABNORMALITIES**
>
> Hole (defect)
>
> Narrowing causing obstruction (stenosis)
>
> Underdevelopment or absence (hypoplasia/atresia)
>
> Wrong connection (transposition/inversion/anomalous connection)

types of lesion into categories and identify patterns, as well as point out different names for the same lesion. Syndromes are then made up of these fundamental building blocks.

Defects

Defects, or holes, can be associated with three different levels in the heart (Box 2–2). They can be associated with the atrial septum, the ventricular septum, or the arterial level. For each of these levels, the physiology within the group is very similar, and there are a limited number of anatomic variants.

Atrial Septal Defects

Most atrial septal defects are classified into four main groups depending on the location of the defect: secundum, primum, sinus venosus, and coronary sinus (Table 2–1 and Fig. 2–1). These names are related to events and structures in the embryological development of the heart. The first atrial

BOX 2-2
THREE LEVELS OF DEFECTS

Atrial septum

  Secundum

  Primum

  Sinus venosus

  Coronary sinus

Ventricular septum

  Perimembranous

  Supracristal

  Malalignment

  Muscular

  Atrioventricular septal defect

Arterial

  Patent ductus arteriosus

  Aortopulmonary window

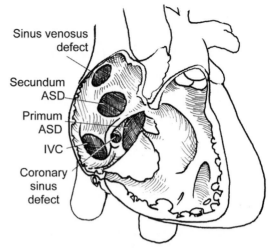

Figure 2–1. The most common types of atrial septal defects (ASDs) are the secundum and primum atrial septal defects, located in the central portion of the atrial septum and toward the tricuspid valves, respectively. Less common is the sinus venosus defect, which is most commonly located near the junction with the superior vena cava as shown here, but it may also be located near the junction with the inferior vena cava (IVC). The least common is an atrial septal defect associated with the coronary sinus.

septum (septum primum) to develop arises from the endocardial cushion and starts at the atrioventricular valves, growing toward the free wall of the combined atrium. Later, there is a second septum (septum secundum), which starts at the free wall of the atrium and grows toward the septum primum. The veins returning to the heart in the embryo combine to form a small chamber (sinus venosus) just before entering the atria. These structures give their names to the most common types of atrial septal defects.

Secundum defects are in the middle of the atrial septum (septum secundum) and are not usually associated with other defects. Primum atrial septal defects are lo-

cated lower in the atrial septum (septum primum) and involve the mitral and tricuspid annuli. Primum defects are part of a constellation of defects that, in its complete form, is called atrioventricular septal defect. The full expression of this syndrome is also called either endocardial cushion defect or atrioventricular canal. It is discussed in detail in the section on Syndromes, but it is worth noting here that, in contrast to secundum defects, primum defects are always associated with abnormalities of the relationship of the tricuspid and mitral valves and a cleft of the anterior mitral leaflet.

The last relatively common form of atrial septal defect is the sinus venosus defect, which is usually located high in the atrial septum, adjacent to the superior vena cava. In this location, it is frequently associated with an anomalous right upper pulmonary vein. A less common location is low in the atrial septum, close to the inferior vena cava. Finally, for completeness, a quite rare form of atrial septal defect is located close to the coronary sinus.

Ventricular Septal Defects

There are five main types of ventricular septal defects (Table 2–2 and Fig. 2–2),

Table 2–1. Types of Atrial Septal Defects

Location	Name	Alternate Names
Midseptum	Secundum ASD	None
Near AV valves	Primum ASD	Partial AV canal
Near SVC	Sinus venosus ASD	None
Near IVC	Sinus venosus ASD	None
Near coronary sinus	Coronary Sinus ASD	None

ASD, atrial septal defect; AV, atrioventricular; IVC, inferior vena cava; SVC, superior vena cava.

Table 2–2. Types of Ventricular Septal Defects

Location	Name	Alternate Names
Outlet, below crista	Perimembranous VSD	Membranous, infracristal (subaortic)
Outlet, above crista	Supracristal VSD	Infundibular, conus (subpulmonary)
Outlet, with malalignment	Malalignment VSD	Part of Tetralogy, double outlet, etc.
Muscular septum	Muscular VSD	Trabecular
AV valves	Atrioventricular SD	Endocardial cushion, AV canal, inlet

AV, atrioventricular; SD, septal defect; VSD, ventricular septal defect.

which can be associated with three areas: the atrioventricular valves, outlet, or muscular portions of the septum.

The most common type of ventricular septal defect is the perimembranous ventricular septal defect. It is located in the membranous part of the ventricular septum, which separates the left ventricular outflow tract from the right ventricle and the right atrium. Because of this location, it is one of the "outlet" types of defects. It is usually located on the portion of the membranous septum adjacent to the muscular septum, and it can involve part of the muscular septum as well. Other names for the same type of defect are membranous, infracristal, and subaortic ventricular septal defect, although the latter is to be avoided for reasons that

are explained shortly. Two anatomic features are worth noting. First, the defects may undermine part of the aortic annulus, resulting in aortic insufficiency in 2% to 5% of patients. Second, it is possible to have a defect from the left ventricular outflow tract to the right atrium, because part of the membranous septum separates the left ventricular outflow tract from the right atrium. Some authors would not call this latter type of defect a ventricular septal defect, because it connects the atrium and ventricle.

The second type of outflow ventricular septal defect to be considered is the supracristal defect. It is so named because it occurs above the crista ventricularis, which is a band of muscle in the posterior right ventricular outflow tract. In contrast, the

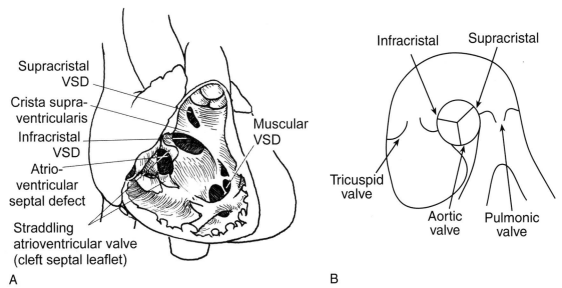

A   B

Figure 2–2. The location of some common types of ventricular septal defects (VSDs) are shown in an anterior drawing (A) and in the short-axis cross-section schematic (B). The supracristal VSD is located immediately below the pulmonic valve and adjacent to the aortic annulus but above the bundle of muscle called the crista ventricularis. The infracristal VSD (also called the perimembranous or membranous VSD) is below the crista ventricularis, but still adjacent to the aortic annulus. The atrioventricular type of ventricular septal defect involves the tricuspid and mitral annuli, whereas the muscular VSD can be located anywhere in the muscular septum, although some locations are more common than others (see text). Not illustrated is the malalignment VSD.

perimembranous defect can also be called an infracristal defect, because it is just below the crista ventricularis. Other names for the supracristal ventricular septal defect are subpulmonary, infundibular, or conal ventricular septal defect.

The supracristal defect is located just below the pulmonary valve and also below the aortic valve. Because of the location of this ventricular septal defect, the disturbed flow may be mistaken for pulmonic stenosis. The terms "subpulmonary" and "subaortic" can be confusing terms because both the supracristal and perimembranous defects are, in fact, both subaortic and subpulmonary, with the supracristal defect closer to the pulmonic valve. This is important to know both for the anatomic relationships and for the association with other defects. The supracristal ventricular septal defect is associated with aortic insufficiency, with a higher incidence than the perimembranous defect, occurring in 5% to 7% of patients with this defect. Because the supracristal defect is also located below the aortic valve and is, in fact, associated with a higher incidence of aortic insufficiency than the perimembranous defect, I prefer to avoid the terms subpulmonary and subaortic defects because of the confusion this can cause.

The last type of "outlet" ventricular septal defect is in a location similar to the preceding two types, called the malalignment ventricular septal defect. It is always associated with overriding of one of the great arteries relative to the ventricular septum, hence its name. The location of this type of ventricular septal defect is anterior and superior relative to the perimembranous defect. However, it is quite close to the perimembranous defect in location. Malalignment defects are always part of a combination of defects in a syndrome, with important management and surgical consequences.

The second location for ventricular septal defects is muscular. This can be in various parts of the muscular septum, including the inlet, outlet, or trabecular portions of the muscular septum. Common sites for small defects are the apex of the right ventricle and at the anterior junction with the right ventricular free wall.

The final location for ventricular septal defects is directly associated with the atrioventricular valves and is of the atrioventricular septal defect type. This is always part of a combination of abnormalities, just like the primum atrial septal defect. This type of lesion is located between the mitral and tricuspid valves and is always associated with abnormalities of the relationship of the two valves and a cleft in the anterior mitral leaflet. The complete syndrome consists of primum atrial septal defect, ventricular septal defect of this type, cleft mitral valve, and the associated abnormalities of the tricuspid valve. This is discussed in further detail in the section on Syndromes.

Arterial Level

Defects at the arterial level are primarily of two types. The first is patent ductus arteriosus. This is not properly considered a congenital defect because we all have a patent ductus arteriosus at birth; it is only failure of closure that is pathological. The other defect, aortopulmonary window, is much rarer and occurs as a hole between the ascending aorta and the main pulmonary artery. It is a defect of septation of the truncus arteriosus. This is discussed in further detail under Division of the Truncus Arteriosus.

Stenoses

As a mnemonic aid, stenoses can be associated with the four major cardiac valves. Stenosis of the atrioventricular valves is not common but can occur congenitally as mitral or tricuspid stenosis.

Stenosis of the semilunar valves is a more complex problem, because the lesions can occur at one of four different levels (Tables 2–3 and 2–4). We can consider the narrowings associated with each semilunar valve as occurring at one of four levels: under, at, over, or distal to the valve. The first three can also be called subvalvular, valvular, and supravalvular stenoses, respectively.

For the aortic valve, the subvalvular ste-

Table 2–3. Types of Stenoses Associated With the Aortic Valve

Location	Type	Names
Below valve	Discrete AS	Subaortic stenosis (membranous)
	Muscular	Hypertrophic obstructive cardiomyopathy
At valve	Valvular	Valvular AS (tri-, bi-, and unicuspid)
Above valve	Diffuse narrowing	Supravalvular AS (Williams syndrome)
Distal	Aortic arch	Infantile coarctation, preductal hypoplasia
	Next to duct	Juvenile coarctation, juxtaductal

AS, aortic stenosis.

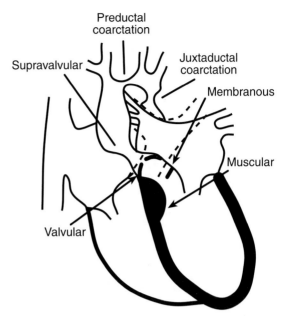

Figure 2–3. Representation of all levels of stenosis that can be associated with the aortic valve, although not at the same time. Illustrated here are the subvalvular membrane, subvalvular muscular obstruction, valvular stenosis, supravalvular stenosis, preductal hypoplasia, and coarctation of the juxtaductal type. Note that the subvalvular membrane is actually usually located on the ventricular septal side of the left ventricular outflow tract but is shown opposite here for clarity.

nosis can be either muscular or discrete. If it is muscular, it causes somewhat different physiology because of the dynamic obstruction. It almost always develops later in life, although it is often inherited. The discrete form is caused by a fibrous membrane in the left ventricular outflow tract (Fig. 2–3).

Valvular aortic stenosis is often associated with a bicuspid or unicuspid aortic valve. Supravalvular aortic stenosis is frequently associated with Williams syndrome. Finally, the distal stenosis is a narrowing occurring in the aorta far from the aortic valve. This is represented by coarctation of the aorta, which is usually located in the aortic arch or just after it (see Fig. 2–3).

Coarctation is often confusing, but when we consider the clinical presentation, most cases fall into two categories. Those that present in childhood are usually a discrete narrowing just beyond the left subclavian artery. This may be before, after, or just adjacent to the remnant of the ductus arteriosus (pre-, post-, or juxtaductal). The other type presents in infancy, with heart failure or shock, and these cases are almost always associated with a more generalized hypoplasia of the aortic arch (preductal segmental tubular hypoplasia). It is perhaps helpful to think of these two groups as the juvenile and infantile types of coarctation because, for practical purposes, the time of presentation is usually different.

For the pulmonic valve, we can make the same subdivision: subpulmonic (or infundibular) stenosis, valvular pulmonic stenosis, and the distal form called peripheral pulmonic stenosis (Fig. 2–4 and see Table 2–4). The supravalvular form is unusual as an isolated defect and is usually grouped as a diagnosis with peripheral pulmonic stenosis, although it can occur as a result of prior pulmonary artery banding (see Physiology). Subpulmonic stenosis is usually muscular, because the right ventricular outflow tract

Table 2–4. Types of Stenoses Associated With the Pulmonary Valve

Location	Type	Names
Below valve	Muscular	Infundibular, muscular bands
At valve	Valvular	Valvular pulmonary stenosis
Above valve	Diffuse narrowing	Pulmonary artery stenosis
Distal	Branches	Peripheral pulmonary stenosis

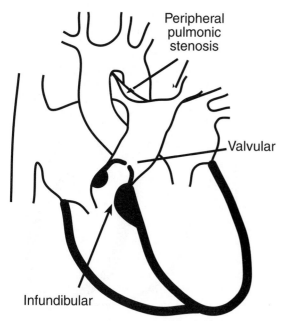

Peripheral pulmonic stenosis

Valvular

Infundibular

Figure 2–4. Representation of levels of stenosis commonly associated with the pulmonic valve. The subvalvular type is also called infundibular. Isolated supravalvular stenosis is exceedingly rare, so it is not illustrated here.

is entirely composed of myocardium, whereas portions of the left ventricular outflow tract are composed of fibrous tissue.

Hypoplasia/Atresia

Hypoplasia (underdevelopment) and atresia (absence) can be associated with each of the cardiac valves and with both of the ventricles. Atresia of any of the valves is a major defect and cannot occur without the presence of other defects or consequences, which are described further under Role of Flow in the Development of Cardiac Structures. Similarly, hypoplasia of one of the ventricles always occurs in conjunction with (and usually because of) other major defects, as is explained in Role of Flow in the Development of Cardiac Structures. It is important to note that confusion is sometimes caused by the use of the term "hypoplastic left ventricle" to refer to an anatomic finding of a small left ventricle and at other times to refer to the syndrome that is better known as "hypoplastic left heart" (see Syndromes). In this book, to avoid confusion,

the terms "hypoplastic left ventricle" and "hypoplastic right ventricle" will always refer to the anatomic finding, with or without the other elements of the syndromes, which are referred to as "hypoplastic left heart" or "hypoplastic right heart."

Wrong Connections

The final category of isolated anatomic defects is wrong connections. These can, in principle, occur at three different levels where connections are located: arterioventricular, ventriculoatrial, and atriovenous. These wrong connections can consist of switching of the normal connections or displacement of the connections (Box 2–3). At the arterioventricular level, switching of the pulmonary artery and aorta results in transposition of the great vessels (Fig. 2–5), whereas displacement results in a double-outlet ventricle. If the vessels come out of the right ventricle, it is called double-outlet right ventricle (Fig. 2–6). If the vessels come out of the left ventricle, it is called double-outlet left ventricle. Both forms of displacement occur exclusively in association with either malalignment ventricular septal defects or absent ventricular septum, so they

---

BOX 2–3
TYPES OF WRONG CONNECTIONS

Switching
  Arterioventricular
    Transposition of the great arteries
  Ventriculoatrial
    Ventricular inversion
  Atriovenous
    (Total anomalous pulmonary veins)
Displacement
  Arterioventricular
    Double-outlet right/left ventricle
  Ventriculoatrial
    Double-inlet right/left ventricle
  Atriovenous
    Total anomalous pulmonary veins

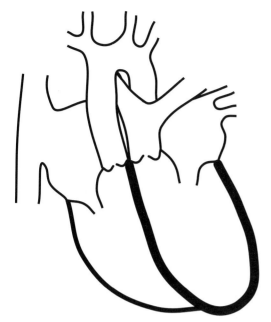

Figure 2–5. Transposition of the great arteries, showing the pulmonary artery exiting from the left ventricle and the aorta exiting from the right ventricle. If there are no other associated lesions, the infant is dependent on ductus arteriosus flow for systemic oxygenation.

cannot properly be considered isolated defects. It is also common for there to be concomitant transposition of the great vessels, and sometimes pulmonic stenosis as well.

Switching at the atrioventricular level is commonly combined with a switch at the arterial level as well, resulting in ventricular inversion. This combination produces no shunts but subjects the anatomic right ventricle to systemic pressures and is often associated with conduction abnormalities such as third-degree heart block. The condition of displaced connections between the atria and ventricles is called double-inlet right ventricle if both the mitral and tricuspid valves empty into the right ventricle, whereas that in which both valves empty into the left ventricle is called double-inlet left ventricle. Just as for the double-outlet defects, the double-inlet defects do not occur in isolation; ventricular septal defect or an absent ventricular septum is mandatory, and complex associations are common.

At the venous level, complete switching does not occur, but wrong connections are represented by partial or total anomalous pulmonary veins, which have some or all of the pulmonary veins draining into the right atrium (Fig. 2–7). In more complex forms of congenital heart disease, there may be atrial isomerism (switching of the atria) or two atria of mirror-image morphologies, and this can be associated with abnormalities of the connection of the systemic venous return as well.

With the congenital defects having to do with wrong connections, there is often confusion about the terminology for the cardiac structures. The most complex congenital lesions involve malposition of the cardiac structures, and this leads to confusion about the nomenclature. Appendix B contains a more detailed overview of the types and nomenclature of cardiac malposition defects. The following guidelines should help in most situations.

First, it is worth noting that the terms "right" and "left" as in "right ventricle" and "left atrium" are anatomic terms and have nothing to do with either the location in the patient (i.e., the right or left side) or the physiological function (systemic or pulmonary). Understanding this fact will avert

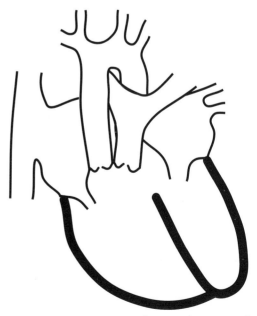

Figure 2–6. Double-outlet right ventricle accompanied by transposition of the great arteries and a malalignment ventricular septal defect. Displacement of the great vessels is always associated with either a malalignment ventricular septal defect or absent ventricular septum.

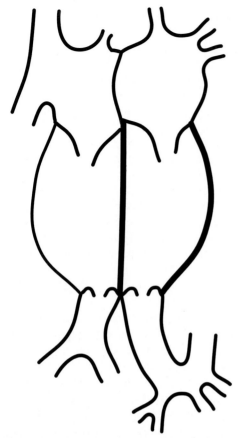

Figure 2–7. "Physiological" diagram of the heart, with the atria above and the ventricles below, illustrating partial anomalous pulmonary veins. Note that there are three pulmonary veins emptying into the left atrium (above right) and one emptying into the right atrium (above left), along with the superior vena cava and inferior vena cava.

called the truncus arteriosus, and the valve is called the truncal valve.

The ventricles are named based on their morphology, not their connections or location. The anatomic right ventricle has heavy trabeculations and generally has a muscular band from the septum to the free wall (the moderator band). The apex usually does not extend as far out toward the cardiac apex as does the anatomic left ventricle. If each ventricle has only one atrioventricular valve, the valve associated with the right ventricle is the tricuspid. The tricuspid valve is located closer to the cardiac apex, except in endocardial cushion defects (see Syndromes).

The anatomic left ventricle has smoother trabeculations and may have fibrous bands crossing it (false tendons), but does not have a moderator band. The apex extends further toward the cardiac apex. If there are distinct atrioventricular valves for each ventricle, the left ventricle's valve is the mitral valve and is located farther from the ventricular apex, except as noted previously.

The atria can be difficult to distinguish on echocardiography, but the most prominent feature is the atrial appendage. This is long and narrow on the left atrium but short and wide on the right atrium. It is often easier to determine lung morphology from the chest x-ray film, and atrial morphology follows lung morphology. This is discussed further in Appendix B.

In this context, it is appropriate to briefly discuss what is meant by the term "dextrocardia." Dextrocardia indicates only that the heart is in the right half of the thorax. It does not imply anything about the relative location of the ventricles or other cardiac structures. Conceptually, it is helpful to distinguish the following three major forms of dextrocardia because this will influence the echocardiographic technique used to obtain standard views (Table 2–5). The first is mirror-image dextrocardia, in which all of the structures are exact mirror images of what they would normally be. This means that the apex is pointed toward the right, but the right ventricle is still located anteriorly and the left ventricle posteriorly. The second is dextrorotation, which can be visualized as the apex of the heart being rotated to-

serious confusion. This means that there is no contradiction or paradox in a patient having two right atria or a right ventricle that is located to the left of the left ventricle and pumps oxygenated blood out the aorta to the systemic circulation.

With this in mind, we can start with the great vessels. These are named for the location to which they lead. This means that the vessel that connects to the aortic arch is called the aorta, and the vessel that connects to the pulmonary arteries is called the main pulmonary artery. Similarly, the semilunar valve at the base of the aorta is the aortic valve, and the valve at the base of the main pulmonary artery is the pulmonic valve. If it is not possible to identify two separate great vessels, the one vessel is

Table 2–5. Types of Dextrocardia

Type	Cardiac Apex	Right Ventricle	Left Ventricle
Mirror image	Right	Anterior	Posterior
Dextrorotation	Right	Posterior	Anterior
Dextroposition	Left	Anterior	Posterior

ward the right from its normal leftward position. This results in the right ventricle being located posteriorly and the left ventricle anteriorly. The third is dextroposition, in which the cardiac structures are just shifted into the right chest without any rotation in the structures. This means that the apex of the heart is still pointed toward the left and the left ventricle is still posterior. For a more detailed discussion of dextrocardia syndromes, see Appendix B.

The echocardiographic consequences can be illustrated by considering how we would obtain a view of all four chambers from the apex. Both the mirror-image dextrocardia heart and the dextroverted heart would be imaged from the right side, but with the transducer orientation reversed relative to each other if we wish to have the same orientation of the right and left ventricles. The dextropositioned heart would have the apical views from the subcostal position.

SYNDROMES

Another area that often causes confusion is syndromes, or predictable combinations of congenital heart defects. The word "syndrome" comes from the Greek *syn,* meaning together and *drome,* meaning run. Thus, it refers to several defects that "run together" or are often found together.

Knowledge of syndromes is extremely important for the performance of a practical echocardiographic examination because the presence of one part of a recognized syndrome should alert the examiner to the possibility or necessity of the other parts being present, and the examination can be directed to identifying and quantifying the other components. Similarly, the absence of an expected combination could alert the examiner to the presence of another defect or an error in the original diagnosis.

Many of the most common syndromes can be grouped together based on an elementary understanding of the development of the heart. In fact, three embryological principles can be used to understand most of the syndromes that will be seen in clinical practice: the function of the endocardial cushion, division of the truncus arteriosus, and role of flow in the development of cardiac structures. Although these embryological principles are based on current understanding of cardiac development, they should not be considered literally true but as rather mnemonic aids to understanding syndromes. Each of these is discussed next.

Many other syndromes are associated with prominent defects outside of the cardiovascular system and have specific names, often of the individuals who gave the first clear description of the syndrome. Some of these syndromes are discussed at the end of this section.

Function of the Endocardial Cushion

The endocardial cushion is a small piece of tissue in the center of the developing heart, which contributes to the formation of several cardiac structures. It is quite literally at the heart of the heart, located between the developing mitral and tricuspid valves and at the juncture of the atrial and ventricular septa (Fig. 2–8). It contributes to the development of the atrial septum, ventricular septum, mitral valve, and tricuspid valve.

The atrial septum develops first from the back wall of the atrium toward the atrioventricular valves, leaving a defect close to the valves. This defect is then closed by a ridge of tissue growing upward from the endocardial cushion. Similarly, the ventricular septum develops from a ridge in the ventricular wall, leaving a defect near the atrioventricular valves, which is also closed by a ridge of tissue arising from the endocardial cushion.

The endocardial cushion contributes to the continuity of the anterior mitral valve leaflet, which actually starts out as two parts that later fuse. Similarly, the septal leaflet of the tricuspid valve starts out as two parts, which fuse as a result of endocar-

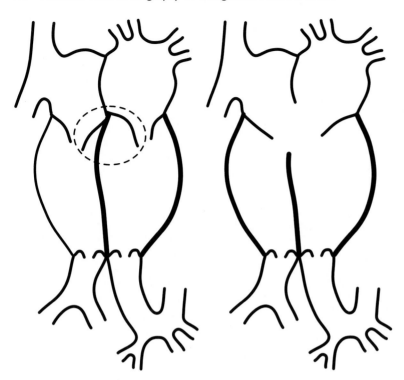

Figure 2–8. Diagram illustrating the structures that are derived from the endocardial cushion. Left, "Normal" view of this physiological/anatomic diagram; the dotted line encircles the structures that are derived from the endocardial cushion in the center of the heart. Right, The result if none of the structures derived from the endocardial cushion develop. There is a defect in the center of the heart, encompassing the lower portion of the atrial septum (primum atrial septal defect), the inlet portion of the ventricular septum, and both of the atrioventricular valves, functionally resulting in a single, bridging valve.

dial cushion development. The portion of the annulus of both valves that separates the valves also develops from the endocardial cushion and results in a slight offset of the valves relative to each other. This can be seen in the four-chamber views as the tricuspid valve being closer to the apex of the heart than the mitral valve (see Fig. 2–8).

We can now consider what would happen if the endocardial cushion failed to perform these functions. We would expect a defect in the atrial septum adjacent to the atrioventricular valves (a primum atrial septal defect); a defect in the ventricular septum, also adjacent to the atrioventricular valves (an inlet type of ventricular septal defect); a split in the anterior mitral valve leaflet (usually called a cleft anterior mitral leaflet); a split in the septal tricuspid leaflet; and a gap in the tricuspid and mitral valve annuli, joining the two valves into one large atrioventricular valve (Fig. 2–9). This is, in fact, the description of the fully developed atrioventricular septal defect, also called endocardial cushion defect or complete atrioventricular canal.

Note that a patient can have a secundum atrial septal defect and a perimembranous ventricular septal defect and still not have an atrioventricular septal defect, because the types of defects in the atrioventricular septal defect are very specific. Because the prognosis, and especially the surgical approach to repair, can be very different, it is preferable to specify an atrioventricular septal defect, if that is the case, or the specific types of atrial septal defect and ventricular septal defect, if known. In the prior example, a secundum ventricular septal defect combined with a perimembranous ventricular septal defect would not include a split in the anterior mitral valve leaflet and septal tricuspid leaflet, making repair considerably easier. The anomalous insertion of the chordae also influences the difficulty of repair.

Not all parts of this syndrome must be present in every patient, although some features are always present. The invariant parts are the split (cleft) of the anterior mitral leaflet, the split of the septal leaflet of the tricuspid, and the loss of the offset between the levels of the mitral and tricuspid valves (Table 2–6). This combination, then, represents the minimal manifestation of an endocardial cushion defect. The loss of offset of the atrioventricular valves can

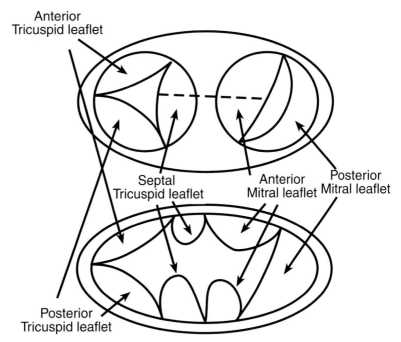

Figure 2–9. Cross-sectional diagram of the atrioventricular valves showing the effects of endocardial cushion defects. The upper diagram is the normal relationship of the mitral and tricuspid valves; the dotted line shows an imaginary cut that yields the appearance below, which is that of the complete endocardial cushion defect. The division of the two valves from each other does not occur, and there is splitting of the anterior leaflet of the mitral valve as well as the septal leaflet of the tricuspid valve.

almost always be identified echocardiographically, as can the split of the anterior mitral valve leaflet. The septal tricuspid leaflet is usually poorly seen; therefore, this part of the syndrome is difficult to identify.

In addition to the unchanging parts of the syndrome, a patient may have only the primum atrial septal defect or the inlet ventricular septal defect or may have both, which would comprise the "complete" syndrome (see Table 2–6). The examiner should look carefully for ventricular septal and atrial septal defects or the physiological consequences of such defects if loss of offset of the atrioventricular valves or a split anterior mitral leaflet is identified.

One other factor that is of major importance in the evaluation of some of these patients is the insertion of the atrioventricular valve chordae. When the ventricular septal defect is large, the chordae of the atrioventricular valves can insert correctly into their respective ventricles, be attached to the crest of the ventricular septum along the defect, or even insert into the wrong ventricle. Each of these added levels of complexity makes repair of the atrioventricular valve more difficult or, in some cases, even impossible. These details of chordae insertion are better seen with echocardiography than with any other technique, although transesophageal studies may be necessary in some situations.

Table 2–6. Combinations of Endocardial Cushion Defects

Name	VSD	ASD	Cleft AMVL, Loss of Offset MV-TV
Cleft AMVL	No	No	Yes
Primum ASD	No	Yes	Yes
VSD-AVSD type	Yes	No	Yes
AVSD	Yes	Yes	Yes

AMVL, anterior mitral valve leaflet; ASD, atrial septal defect; AVSD, atrioventricular septal defect; MV, mitral valve; TV, tricuspid valve; VSD, ventricular septal defect.

Division of the Truncus Arteriosus

The pulmonary artery and aorta develop from a single artery leaving the heart in the fetus. This artery is called the truncus arteriosus, and an understanding of how it develops into two separate arteries helps us understand the abnormal development of a number of cardiac syndromes.

The truncus arteriosus overrides the ventricular septum and branches into the main pulmonary artery and ascending aorta. It is eventually divided by a septum, which separates the ascending aorta from the pulmonary artery and connects with the ventricular septum, closing the ventricular septal defect. An interesting and important detail is that this septum has to undergo a 180-degree twist to make the connections correctly (Fig. 2–10). This is because the pulmonary arteries are posteriorly directed, whereas the right ventricle is actually anterior. Similarly, the ascending aorta is anterior, whereas the left ventricle is posterior.

With this development in mind, perhaps the easiest defect to imagine is if the septation occurs but without the twist. In this case, the anterior (right) ventricle will be attached to the anterior artery (ascending aorta), whereas the posterior ventricle (left) will be attached to the posterior artery (pulmonary). This is the situation with transposition of the great arteries. Another simple defect to imagine is an incomplete septation. In this case, there will be a defect between the aorta and pulmonary artery, which is called an aortopulmonary window. Neither of these can properly be considered a syndrome because they are actually just isolated defects, but they illustrate the simplest cases of defects of division of the truncus arteriosus.

The most common example of a syndrome related to the division of the truncus arteriosus can be imagined if we consider what would happen if the dividing septum in the truncus were to be displaced anteriorly. The pulmonary artery and pulmonic valve would become smaller as a result of this anterior displacement, and the aorta and aortic valve would become larger and override the ventricular septum, because the size that was gained would be anterior. There would be a disturbance of the connection between the ventricular septum and the septation of the truncus because of the displacement, resulting in a malalignment type of ventricular septal defect. This combination of overriding aorta, ventricular septal defect, and pulmonic stenosis is known as tetralogy of Fallot, although "tetrad of Fallot" would be linguistically more correct. It is called a tetralogy rather than a trilogy because of the inevitable right ventricular hypertrophy,

which became part of the syndrome as described in 1888.

Other combinations are also possible, especially when we add displacement of the entire truncus anteriorly or posteriorly. These include double-outlet right ventricle, double-outlet left ventricle, and many others, some bearing specific names. These are outlined in Table 2–7.

Role of Flow in the Development of Cardiac Structures

Blood flow is critical to the development of cardiac structures in the fetal period. If the flow through a cardiac structure is limited or absent, that structure cannot develop normally. If this restriction occurs early enough during the development, that structure and the structures "downstream" will become small (hypoplastic) or even completely absent (atretic) (Fig. 2–11).

This means that a single defect, such as mitral atresia, will provoke a cascade of consequences, because all of the structures that are downstream will not receive sufficient blood flow to develop normally (Fig. 2–12). In this example, there would be hypoplasia of the left ventricle, aortic valve, and ascending aorta. The distal aorta would not be affected because it would receive blood flow through the ductus arteriosus. The resulting syndrome is hypoplastic left heart syndrome. A similar sequence of events can occur on the right side of the heart. If there is tricuspid atresia, it would trigger hypoplasia of the right ventricle, pulmonic valve, and main pulmonary artery (Fig. 2–13). Of note is that both of the combinations described, as well as all of the combinations caused by failure of adequate flow to one side of the heart, result in a dependence on flow through the open ductus arteriosus for an adequate circulation. This is discussed in more detail later.

Defects that are further downstream will also cause side effects, but the effects proximal and distal to the primary defect will be different. A prime example is severe pulmonary stenosis or atresia. Because there is no or little flow through the pulmonic valve, the main pulmonary artery is also hypoplas-

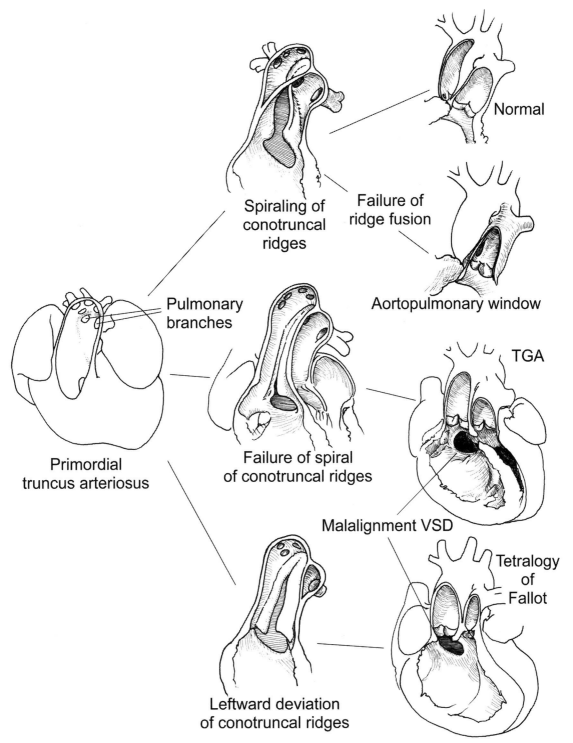

Figure 2–10. Division of the truncus arteriosus. The pulmonary arteries exit from the posterior portion of the truncus, whereas the right ventricle is anterior (left center). This means that the septation must undergo a 180-degree twist to make the correct connections (top branches). Abnormalities of the position, degree of twist of the septation, and degree of fusion can cause a number or syndromes, including tetralogy of Fallot, transposition of the great arteries (TGA), and aortopulmonary window, among others (see text). VSD, ventricular septal defect.

Table 2–7. Defects Related to Truncal Position and Septation

Name	Truncal Position	Septum Position	Septum Twist
TGA	Normal	Normal	None
TOF	Normal	Anterior	Yes
DORV	Anterior	Normal	Yes
DORV + TGA	Anterior	Normal	None
DORV + TGA + PS	Anterior	Posterior	None
DOLV	Posterior	Normal	Yes
DOLV + TGA	Posterior	Normal	None

DOLV, double-outlet left ventricle; DORV, double-outlet right ventricle; PS, pulmonary stenosis; TGA, transposition of great arteries; TOF, tetralogy of Fallot.

tic, as expected. The right ventricle is exposed to less flow as well and fails to develop normally. What is different, though, is that the right ventricle is exposed to a pressure load at the same time as there is little flow. As a result, in addition to small chamber size, the wall becomes hypertrophic. The result is a combination of pulmo-

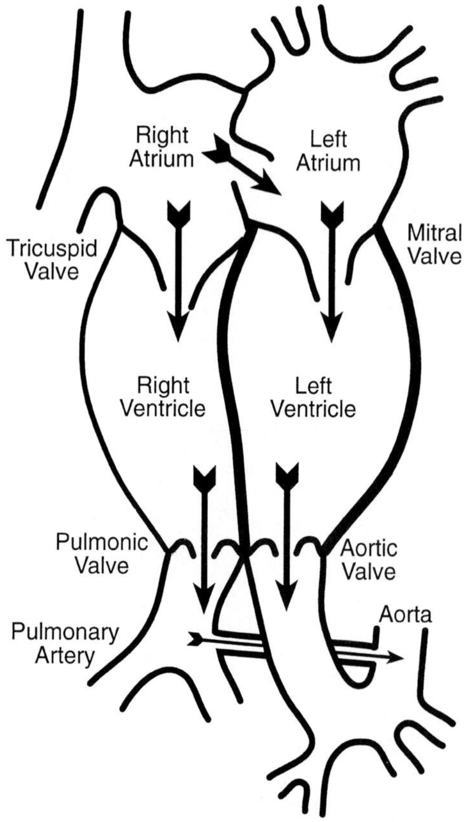

Figure 2–11. Illustration of the flow patterns in the normal fetal heart. Because flow is necessary for normal development, disruption in the flow at any stage will cause undergrowth (hypoplasia) or absence (atresia) of structures "downstream" of the disruption.

nary stenosis/atresia, hypoplastic right ventricle, and right ventricular hypertrophy. This combination is sometimes called "peach pit right ventricle" because of the globular shape and heavy trabeculations.

This principle of flow being necessary for the development of cardiac structures also affects the manifestation of other types of syndromes. Tetralogy of Fallot often is accompanied by hypoplasia of the branch pulmonary arteries as well as the main pulmonary artery as a result of the decreased flow. Any form of aortic outflow obstruction may lead to ascending aortic and aortic arch (isthmus) hypoplasia as a consequence of decreased flow.

This cascade effect means that many defects that conceptually are isolated cannot, in fact, occur in isolation. This is because they will influence the development of other structures through their effect on blood flow. We can use this fact in several ways to improve the accuracy of our echocardiographic diagnoses. First, if we know that the defects are related, we should always look for the consequences of a primary defect or the cause of a secondary effect. If we see aortic atresia, we expect the whole ascending aorta to be hypoplastic. If we see a small, hypertrophic right ventricle, we expect to find severe pulmonic stenosis or atresia.

Second, and perhaps more important, is that because we expect certain combinations to occur, if the combination is not present, another defect, perhaps undetected, must exist. A few examples will make this clearer. If we see that the mitral valve is either severely stenotic or atretic and the left ventricle is not hypoplastic, there must be a source for the blood flow that allowed

Figure 2–12. Two examples of the consequences of disruption of the flow on the left side of the heart during fetal life. Left, There is mitral atresia of the "membranous" type (absence of a functioning mitral valve although there is a membrane where the valve should be). This leads to reduced flow through the left ventricle, which is small as a result (hypoplastic). The aortic valve and ascending aorta are also small, but the descending aorta is normal because of flow through the ductus arteriosus. Right, There is aortic stenosis, leading to a small ascending aorta. Note that the descending aorta is normal in size because of ductal flow. If the foramen ovale does not allow flow from left to right, as illustrated, this can also lead to severe enlargement of the left side of the heart. Note that both of these combinations lead to dependence on the ductus arteriosus for adequate circulation.

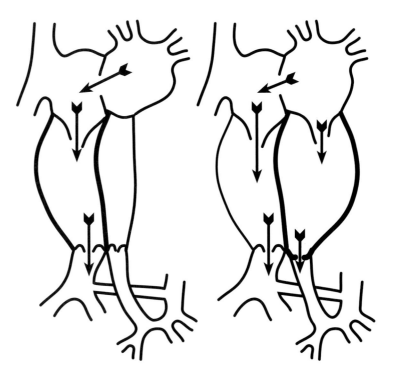

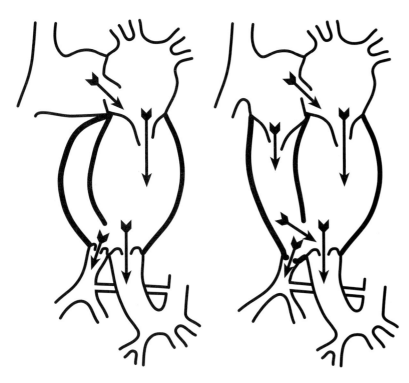

Figure 2–13. Two examples of the consequences of disruption of flow on the right side of the heart during fetal life. Left, There is complete tricuspid atresia (absence of any tricuspid membrane or annulus). This results in undergrowth of the right ventricle and, to a lesser extent, the pulmonary artery, because in this case, a ventricular septal defect allows some flow. Right, There is a severe pulmonic stenosis, which leads to undergrowth (hypoplasia) of the main pulmonary artery and its branches. Note that both of these combinations also lead to dependence on the ductus arteriosus for adequate circulation.

the left ventricle to develop, and it is most likely a ventricular septal defect, even if we have not seen it yet. We can then modify our examination to search actively for the source of blood flow, which we know must be there.

If we have limited views and see that the ascending aorta looks normal in caliber but the left ventricle is severely hypoplastic, we know that the flow that allowed the ascending aorta to develop must have come from another source, and we would expect to find the aorta arising from the right ventricle.

Similar situations arise on the right side; tricuspid atresia with an almost normal right ventricle suggests the presence of a ventricular septal defect. The net result using this principle, as in using the others, is that it allows us to predict the expected combination of defects and make a more complete and reliable diagnosis as a result.

Other Syndromes

Cardiac defects are common in other congenital syndromes and are the most common organ system affected with congenital defects. Because of this, the number of syndromes that include cardiac defects as possible is very large. It is difficult to classify these because, in many individuals, the cardiac defects do not present until much later in life. Some of the more common of these are listed in Table 2–8.

PHYSIOLOGY

The physiology of congenital heart disease, especially shunts, is often confusing to those who do not deal with it on a regular basis. Fortunately, some very simple principles can be used to sort out the majority of clinically relevant situations. By combining these principles, even the most complex situations can be understood.

A bonus of this physiological approach is that many complex congenital defects reduce to simpler physiological problems, and the consequences to the patient are often determined more by the physiology than the details of anatomy. An example is a patient with no ventricular septum. Although the anatomic distinction between absent ventricular septum (two morphologically distinct ventricles with an atrioventricular valve emptying into each but no ventricular septum) and univentricular heart (no morphological distinction between the ventricles) may be difficult to make based on the structural data available, it is clear that the patient physiologically has only one ventricular cavity. Whether parts of this ventricle are morphologically distinct is critical for the anatomic diagnosis but not for the "physiological" diagnosis.

Volume Versus Pressure Loads

Because the heart is a pump, there are two fundamental aspects to the load to which it is subjected: volume and pressure.

Table 2–8. Other Syndromes

Name	Primary Cardiac Defects	Other Common Defects
Down	VSD, AVSD, primum ASD	Retardation, face, hands
Duchenne's	Cardiomyopathy	Central muscle weakness
Fetal alcohol	VSD	Retardation, face
Holt-Oram	Secundum ASD	Hypoplasia/atresia of radius and thumb
Kartagener's	Mirror image dextrocardia	Bronchiectasis, sinusitis
Marfan	Ascending aortic aneurism, MVP	Tall stature, dislocated lenses
Noonan's	PS, HCM	Neck, face, chest
Rubella	PDA, PPS	Deafness, retardation, eye
Turner's	Coarctation, AS	Neck, chest, infertility
Williams	Supravalvular AS, PS	Retardation, face

AS, aortic stenosis; ASD, atrial septal defect; AVSD, atrioventricular septal defect; HCM, hypertrophic cardiomyopathy; MVP, mitral valve prolapse; PDA, patent ductus arteriosus; PPS, peripheral pulmonic stenosis; PS, pulmonary stenosis; VSD, ventricular septal defect.

The external work performed by the heart is, in fact, defined by the integral of pressure × volume. Because of this, one common way of looking at cardiac function is to plot pressure versus volume, for the so-called pressure-volume loop (Fig. 2–14).

Congenital heart defects can cause an overload that is predominantly volume or pressure or both. The physiological consequences and the anatomic response to the two types of load are quite different. Volume loads cause chamber dilation, whereas pressure loads cause wall hypertrophy. This is true even though there is an intimate relationship between volume and pressure in the heart. The primary type of load determines the primary response. Volume loads result from shunts or valvular regurgitation, whereas pressure loads result from obstruction or increased vascular resistance.

An example of a predominant pressure load is moderate to severe aortic stenosis without significant regurgitation or left ventricular dysfunction (Fig. 2–15). The systolic pressures within the left ventricle will be elevated, and there will be left ventricular hypertrophy. Although wall thickness will be increased, other dimensions will most

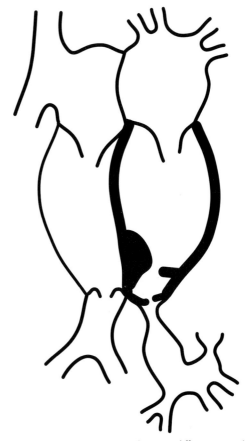

Figure 2–15. Illustration of many different possible causes for pressure (systolic) load on the left side of the heart. Shown are septal hypertrophy causing left ventricular outflow obstruction, a subaortic membrane, valvular aortic stenosis, supravalvular aortic stenosis, and coarctation. Note that the subvalvular membrane is illustrated on the side of the left ventricular outflow tract opposite to where it usually actually occurs and that these lesions do not occur all at once!

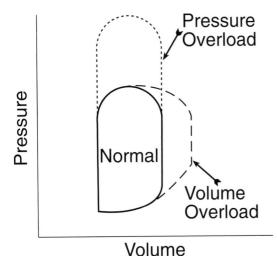

Figure 2–14. Pressure-volume loop relating the pressure in the left ventricle to the volume. The area of the curve is the work performed by the heart. Pressure loads are primarily caused by obstructions, whereas volume loads are caused by shunts and valvular regurgitation. Either type of load results in increased work for the heart.

probably be within normal limits. Pressure loads on the right ventricle are similar in their effects (Fig. 2–16).

The simplest example of an isolated volume load is leakage of one of the valves, or regurgitation. For example, consider aortic regurgitation (Fig. 2–17). If the heart rate and cardiac output are normal, the amount of blood entering the left ventricle through the mitral valve will also be normal, and this will represent the effective forward stroke volume. The amount of blood that fills the ventricle in diastole, however, will be higher, because it will consist of the effective stroke volume plus the regurgitant volume leaking through the aortic valve.

An isolated atrial septal defect will also result in an increase in diastolic filling of the right side of the heart, with resulting right ventricular and atrial dilation, ventricular septal flattening, and paradoxical ventricular septal motion (Fig. 2–18). The paradoxical motion occurs because the septum bulges to the left during diastole secondary to the increased volume and pressure in the right ventricle and to the right during systole because of left ventricular contraction. The increase in diastolic dimension will increase the end-diastolic pressure and also increase the peak systolic pressure caused by increased flow, but the predominant disturbance will still be a volume load with dilation.

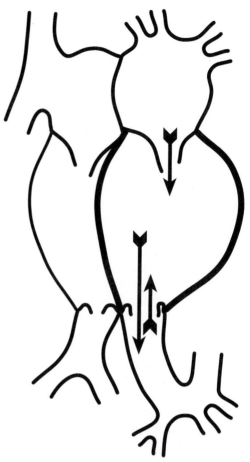

Figure 2–17. Illustration of the volume load of aortic regurgitation. The *arrows* represent the different flows. The flow out the aortic valve during systole is equal to the mitral flow during diastole plus the backward flow through the aortic valve during diastole. This extra volume (diastolic) load causes enlargement of the left ventricular cavity.

Because of the relationship between pressure and volume in the heart, it may be difficult to determine at first whether an extra load is primarily volume or pressure. An example of this is a moderate ventricular septal defect (Fig. 2–19). Because there is a shunt from the left ventricle to the right ventricle, one might be tempted to call this volume (or even pressure) load on the right ventricle. For the purposes of determining the effect on the heart in potentially confusing situations such as this, an additional load on either ventricle that primarily occurs in diastole should be considered a volume load, and a load that occurs primarily in systole should be considered a pressure load (Box 2–4).

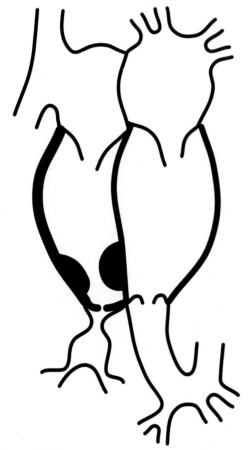

Figure 2–16. Illustration of many different possible causes for pressure (systolic) load on the right side of the heart. Shown are infundibular hypertrophy causing right ventricular outflow obstruction, valvular pulmonic stenosis, supravalvular pulmonic stenosis (rare), and peripheral pulmonic stenosis. Again, these lesions do not occur all at once!

Using this rule, we can see that the additional load on the right ventricle coming from the moderate ventricular septal defect will only be a volume (diastolic) load if it is due to a significant diastolic shunt. As well, a pressure load on the right ventricle will only occur if the ventricular septal defect is so large that there is either equalization of pressures in the two ventricles during systole or such a large shunt that pulmonary artery systolic pressures are elevated. There will, however, be a volume load on the left ventricle and left atrium, which will result in chamber dilation.

Conversely, if there is a significant diastolic shunt, we would expect consequences of a diastolic (volume) load, mainly right ventricular chamber dilation. If there is

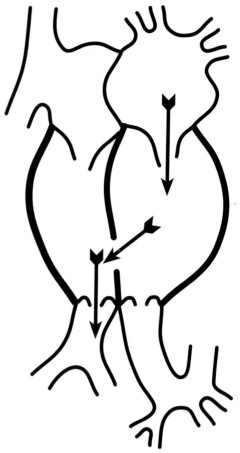

Figure 2–19. An isolated ventricular septal defect results in left-to-right shunting at the ventricular level, with volume (diastolic) overload and resultant dilation of the left atrium and left ventricle. Arrows indicate extra shunt flow.

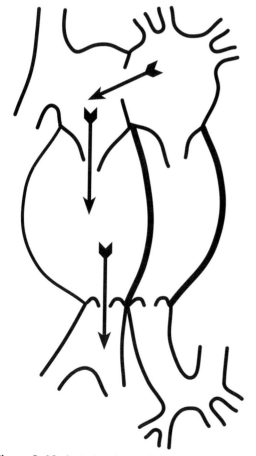

Figure 2–18. An isolated secundum atrial septal defect results in left-to-right shunting at the atrial level, resulting in a volume (diastolic) overload and, therefore, dilation of the atria, right ventricle, and pulmonary artery. Arrows indicate extra shunt flow.

BOX 2–4
TYPES OF VENTRICULAR LOADS

Volume (diastolic) load
Is caused by

  Shunts

  Valvular insufficiency

Results in

  Chamber dilation

Pressure (systolic) load
Is caused by

  Stenoses

  Increased vascular resistance

Results in

  Hypertrophy

equalization of pressures during systole, we would expect right ventricular hypertrophy as a result of this systolic (pressure) load.

We can also link our previous simplified classification of types of congenital heart disease to the type of load that usually predominates. Stenoses distal to the ventricles cause pressure load, with resulting hypertrophy. Defects cause volume loads, whereas atresia causes mixed volume and pressure loading. Displaced connections primarily cause volume loads, and switched connections do not directly cause altered loads at all.

Direction of Shunts

Another potentially confusing topic is the expected direction of a shunt. This is important because, if we find that the direction of the shunt is other than expected, it should lead us to search for the reason for the discrepancy.

To understand the direction of shunts, we can divide defects into those that are restrictive and those that are not restrictive. A restrictive defect is one that restricts the free flow of blood; therefore, there will be a significant pressure gradient across the defect and a high velocity of flow. A nonrestrictive defect does not significantly impede the free flow of blood, resulting in an absence of significant gradient and a low velocity of flow.

For restrictive defects, the direction can be determined by understanding the normal pressure relationships. If there is a restrictive defect, the fundamental relationship of the pressures will not be altered, although the absolute value of the pressure differences may change and the flow will be from the high-pressure chamber to the low-pressure chamber. For nonrestrictive defects, the direction of the shunt will be determined by the relative resistance of the receiving vascular beds, or compliance of the receiving chambers. This is discussed in more detail next.

Restrictive Defects

In the case of an isolated, restrictive defect, the predominant shunt flow will al-

ways be from left to right because the pressures on the left side of the heart are higher than those on the right for each level (Fig. 2–20). This means that if there is an isolated, restrictive atrial septal defect, the predominant shunt flow will be from the left atrium to the right atrium, because the left atrial pressure is higher than right atrial pressure, and this pressure relationship is preserved because of the restrictive nature of the defect. Similarly, for an isolated, restrictive ventricular septal defect, the predominant shunt would be from left to right, because left ventricular pressure is higher than right ventricular pressure. The same logic explains the left-to-right shunt through a patent ductus arteriosus.

It is useful to consider the conditions that could lead to exceptions to these general

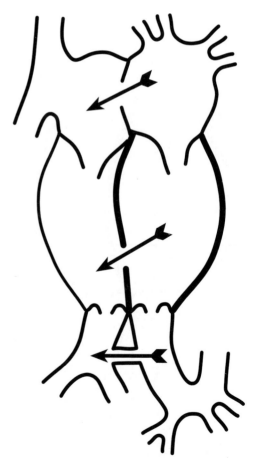

Figure 2–20. For a restrictive defect, the shunt flow will be predominantly left to right at any level in the heart because the left-sided pressures are higher than the right-sided pressures at each level.

rules. At the atrial level, right-to-left shunting would occur even in the presence of a restrictive defect if the right atrial pressure exceeded left atrial pressure. This may occur momentarily during the normal cardiac cycle, leading to a minor right-to-left shunt. It can also occur during physiological maneuvers that raise the right-sided venous pressure, such as Valsalva's maneuver. Any condition that raises the right ventricular end-diastolic pressure (hypertrophy, dilation with failure) can result in an elevated right atrial pressure and right-to-left shunting. Finally, any restriction to outflow from the right atrium (tricuspid stenosis) will also raise its pressure.

At the ventricular level the list is somewhat shorter, although the logic is similar. We may have an elevation of right ventricular diastolic pressures as a result of failure or hypertrophy, which will lead to a momentary right-to-left shunt during diastole. If the right ventricular systolic pressure is elevated above the left ventricular pressures as a result of any type of pulmonic stenosis or pulmonary hypertension, there will be a right-to-left shunt at the ventricular level (Fig. 2–21).

Finally, at the arterial level, right-to-left shunting can occur if there is pulmonary hypertension with pressures exceeding the systemic arterial pressures, regardless of the cause, or if the systemic arterial pressure is lowered for some reason, such as a preductal coarctation of the aorta.

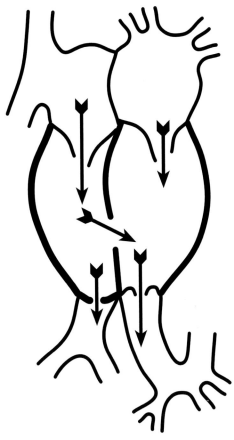

Figure 2–21. If there is an elevation of the right ventricular pressure, for example, resulting from valvular pulmonic stenosis, there can be right-to-left shunting through a ventricular septal defect. This can cause the systemic blood to have a low oxygen saturation, resulting in cyanosis. Arrows indicate blood flow with increased flow due to shunt through tricuspid and aortic valves.

Nonrestrictive Defects

The approach we have followed for restrictive defects is not applicable to nonrestrictive defects. Because there is free flow of blood, there will be no significant pressure difference between the chambers, and we cannot use the pressure difference to determine the predominant direction of shunt. We must use another principle to guide our understanding of the direction of shunting in this situation.

When the pressure in two chambers has been equalized because of a nonrestrictive lesion, there is always bidirectional shunting. The predominant direction of the shunt will be determined by the physiology of the downstream structures: the relative resistance of the downstream vascular beds or the relative compliance of the cardiac chambers. A few examples will make this clearer.

In the case of a nonrestrictive atrial septal defect, there will also be an equalization of pressure between the atria. The flow into the atria will be determined by the relative compliance of the atria. The flow out of the atria during diastole will be determined by the compliance of the receiving ventricular chambers. The chamber with the least resistance to being filled (most compliance) will receive the most blood. In most cases, this will be the right ventricle because it has a thinner wall and is, therefore, less stiff. This will result in a net left-to-right shunt at the atrial level.

In the case of a large ventricular septal defect, pressures in the two ventricular chambers will be equal. Because of this, we cannot determine the direction of the shunt based on the pressure. During diastole, the partitioning of the flow between the two chambers will be dependent on the relative compliance. If the right ventricle is more compliant, the predominant shunt will be left to right because the right ventricle will fill more. During systole, however, because the pressure in both chambers is equal, we would expect the flow out of the ventricles to be determined by the vascular resistance. For example, if the pulmonary vascular resistance is half that of the systemic vascular resistance (it is usually about one-fifth of systemic resistance), we would expect the flow to be twice as high. As a result, there would be a net left-to-right shunt at this level as well.

As in the case of restrictive defects, it is important to consider when our assumptions are not valid. Fortunately, the situations are virtually identical to those for restrictive defects. An atrial level left-to-right shunt will be reduced or reversed by anything that impedes emptying of the right atrium. This includes right ventricular hypertrophy and severe dilation, both of which reduce compliance, and tricuspid stenosis. For a large ventricular septal defect, anything that would increase resistance to flow out of the right ventricle would reduce or even reverse the left-to-right shunt. This includes pulmonary hypertension and any form of pulmonic stenosis.

Consequences of Shunts

Once we have a feeling for the direction and magnitude of a shunt, the next issue is what the consequences of the shunt will be. These can be anatomic responses, physiological effects, or clinical signs, symptoms, or complications. These are all directly related to the direction and magnitude of the shunt.

Chamber Enlargement

The primary change that we expect in shunt lesions is chamber enlargement re-sulting from the extra volume (diastolic) load. What is less clear is which chambers will be affected in the case of a particular congenital defect. A simple rule is that isolated defects before the atrioventricular valves cause right-sided chamber dilation, whereas lesions after the atrioventricular valves cause left-sided chamber dilation. This means that any type of atrial septal defect, without additional defects, will result in right ventricular and right atrial enlargement, whereas all types of isolated ventricular septal defects and arterial level shunts will cause left atrial and left ventricular enlargement (Box 2–5).

One way to understand this is to follow the flow of blood through the heart in various shunt conditions. In the case of an atrial septal defect (Fig. 2–22), the flow through the aortic valve is similar to that returning through the venae cavae, whereas that going through the pulmonic valve is the same as that returning through the pulmonary veins. The pulmonary blood flow, however, is greater than the aortic blood flow by an amount equal to the left-to-right shunt through the atrial septal defect and equal to the tricuspid flow, which is represented by a double arrow in the diagram. This means that all structures that are subjected to, or loaded with, this extra flow should show the effects. In this case, we can see that the right ventricle, right atrium, left atrium, and pulmonary circulation are all affected. In fact, right ventricular and atrial dilation are typical in all forms of atrial

---

BOX 2–5
CONSEQUENCES OF SHUNTS

Atrial level
  Right ventricular enlargement
  Pulmonary artery enlargement
Ventricular level
  Left atrial enlargement
  Left ventricular enlargement
Arterial level
  Left atrial enlargement
  Left ventricular enlargement

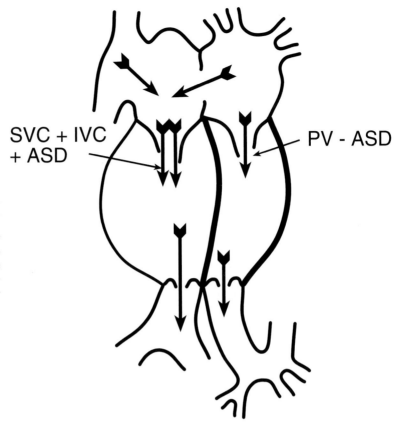

SVC + IVC + ASD

PV - ASD

Figure 2–22. In a nonrestrictive atrial septal defect (ASD), the flow through the tricuspid valve *(double arrows)* is equal to the sum of the combined flow through the atrial septal defect, the superior vena cava (SVC), and the inferior vena cava (IVC). The flow through the pulmonary valve (PV) *(long arrow)* is equal to the tricuspid flow. This increase in flow leads to a volume (diastolic) overload of the right ventricle.

septal defect, and dilation of the pulmonary artery and pulmonary vein can often be identified as well. Left atrial dilation is not pronounced because there is release of the overload into the more compliant right atrium. The left ventricle, aorta, and systemic veins would not normally be affected in an isolated atrial septal defect.

In the case of a moderate ventricular septal defect (Fig. 2–23), the situation is different. The extra flow travels through the left atrium and left ventricle, only passing through the right ventricle during systole and, therefore, not causing right ventricular dilation. Left atrial dilation and left ventricular dilation are prominent, however, in this condition, and dilation of the pulmonary artery can occur.

It is important to realize that significant changes in volume loading are required to cause marked chamber enlargement. In a typical isolated septal defect, the ratio between total pulmonary flow and total systemic flow (also referred to as Qp:Qs) is 1.3 to 2.0, although values greater than 4 are

not uncommon. This means that the flow through the pulmonary circulation, and therefore the load on the affected structures, is 30% to 300% greater than normal.

When the septal defect is not isolated, the situation can be quite different. In the relatively simple case of a ventricular septal defect with pulmonic stenosis, as the stenosis becomes more severe, the magnitude of the shunt will decrease. If the stenosis becomes severe enough to equalize the pressures in the two ventricles, the volume of the shunt may be close to zero. If the stenosis becomes severe enough to raise the pressure in the right ventricle to or above systemic levels, there will be a right-to-left shunt (see Fig. 2–21). The magnitude of this shunt is unlikely to reach the size of the left-to right shunts, however, because this would require the pulmonary vascular plus valvular resistance to be up to four times the systemic resistance. In addition, systemic pressure and flow are more closely regulated by the autonomic system than pulmonary pressure and flow. This means

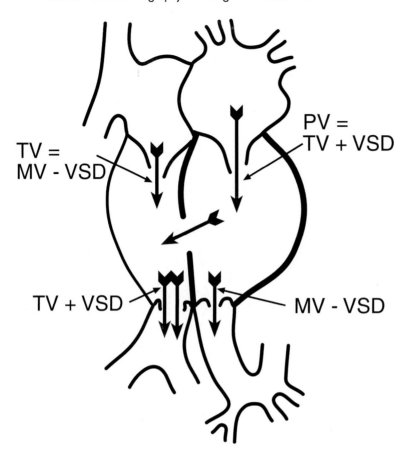

TV =
MV - VSD

PV =
TV + VSD

TV + VSD

MV - VSD

Figure 2–23. The flow through the pulmonic valve (PV) *(double arrows)* in the case of a moderate ventricular septal defect (VSD) is equal to the sum of the tricuspid valve (TV) flow and the ventricular septal defect flow. The mitral valve (MV) flow *(long arrow)* is also increased, resulting in volume (diastolic) overloading of the left ventricle and atrium.

that the degree of chamber dilation that will occur as a consequence of even a severe right-to-left shunting will virtually never be as impressive as that with a left-to-right shunt. The more important sign of right-to-left shunting is cyanosis, discussed later.

A second reason that the chamber enlargement in right-to left shunting will seldom match that in left-to-right shunting is the compliance of the systemic ventricle. The pressures in the systemic side of the heart are normally higher, and this leads to hypertrophy and increased stiffness. This increase in stiffness will restrict the degree of dilation that occurs.

Pressure

With an increase in flow as a result of shunting, there will often be an increase in pressure. It is customary to use a simple "electrical" model for the relationship among flow, pressure, and resistance. In this model, the voltage (V) is equal to the current (I) times the resistance (R), or $V = I \times R$. The analogue for blood flow is that mean pressure (P) is equal to flow (Q) times vascular resistance (VR), or $P = Q \times VR$. This is not actually exactly true, but it is a useful approximation for most clinical situations.

Using this relationship, we can see that if the flow through the pulmonary circulation increases by a factor of two because of a shunt and the pulmonary vascular resistance remains constant, we would expect the mean pressure to increase by a factor of two as well. This rarely occurs, however, because the pulmonary vascular resistance usually falls as the flow increases, and the pressure remains constant because of the reflex control mechanisms to control pulmonary artery pressure. At some point of increasing blood flow, maximal vasodilation will be achieved, and any further increase will result in an increase in pressure.

All of the preceding discussion applies to the relatively acute situation. Chronically, other mechanisms are of importance. In particular, there is a tendency for reflex vasoconstriction if there is significant over-circulation to the lungs. This will cause a further increase in right-sided pressures, which can cause secondary effects such as hypertrophy and reduction of the degree of shunt. The hypertrophy and elevation of pressures can, if severe, even cause right-to-left shunting because of equalization of diastolic or systolic pressures. This vasoconstriction can usually be temporarily relieved with pulmonary vasodilators, such as increasing the inspired oxygen content with an oxygen mask, or intravenous prostacyclin. This can be useful for diagnosing reversible vasoconstriction.

A very serious complication of large left-to-right shunts is the development of irreversible, severe elevation of the pulmonary vascular resistance. If this is sufficiently severe, the right-sided pressures will exceed the left-sided pressures, a condition called Eisenmenger's syndrome when it is the late result of a large shunt. All patients with large left-to-right shunts are at risk for increased pulmonary vascular resistance or even Eisenmenger's syndrome, although the risk is significantly higher in those with high pulmonary pressures since birth and patients with Down syndrome. A possible explanation for the increased risk in those with a large shunt since birth is the increased pulmonary arteriolar smooth muscle all infants have at birth, which normally involutes after birth but may hypertrophy and scar if there is a large shunt.

It should be clear from these points that the right-sided pressures are very important in the assessment of shunt lesions. The right ventricular pressure influences the magnitude of shunt in restrictive lesions but will itself be influenced by the size of the shunt in nonrestrictive lesions. If the right ventricular pressure is sufficiently high because of pulmonary stenosis or elevated pulmonary vascular resistance, the shunt can be so small that it would be difficult to detect with Doppler. High pressures can either be a risk factor for the development of Eisenmenger's syndrome if there is a large shunt or indicate that it has already occurred if the shunt is small or right to

left. These are some of the reasons why assessment of right ventricular systolic pressure using the velocity of tricuspid regurgitation, or pulmonary arterial diastolic pressure using the velocity of pulmonary regurgitation, is of such importance.

Cyanosis

Cyanosis is defined as the finding on physical examination of a blue coloration to the lips, nail beds, or gums. Cyanosis occurs when there is a significant amount of desaturated hemoglobin in the circulation. There are two ways in which this occurs, both of which can be related to shunts. The first is that the blood is never fully saturated with oxygen because of a pulmonary problem. This can be due to a pulmonary diffusion defect, hypoventilation, or intrapulmonary shunting. In severe left-sided heart failure from any cause, there can be a diffusion defect resulting from the interstitial fluid build-up (Box 2–6).

The second is that there is a right-to-left shunt, which means that desaturated blood returning from the body would return to the systemic circulation. Note that this will not occur to a significant degree with isolated, restrictive defects; therefore, a patent ductus, ventricular septal defect, or atrial septal defect is not normally cyanotic defects when occurring alone. This is because of the normal pressure relationships in the heart, which will result in left-to-right shunting. If we see cyanosis or echocardiographic evidence for right-to-left shunting, we must

---

BOX 2–6
CAUSES OF CYANOSIS

Pulmonary
  Diffusion defect
  Hypoventilation
  Intrapulmonary shunt
Cardiac
  Right-to-left shunt
  Cardiac failure (diffusion)
Noncardiopulmonary

look for another defect, or defects, that would account for either equalization of pressures or increase of right-sided pressures higher than the left-sided pressures. For a discussion of the clinical differentiation between pulmonary and cardiac causes of cyanosis in the newborn, see Pulmonary Versus Cardiac Disease in Chapter 4.

Cyanotic lesions can result in quite severe desaturation, but there are other risks as well. The desaturation itself can cause decreased exercise tolerance, and there is often a compensatory increase in the number of red cells in the blood to compensate for the decreased oxygen carried by the blood. If the number of red cells increases too much, the viscosity of the blood may increase to a point where this also results in increased coagulability and slowed circulation, causing thrombotic disorders.

Embolization

Whenever there is a right-to-left shunt, there is a risk of right-to-left embolization, also called paradoxical embolization, because the source is in the right circulation whereas the results are on the left. This is because the lungs provide a significant filtering function in addition to exchanging gases. When this "filter" is bypassed because of a right-to-left shunting, a number of complications are much more likely.

In the course of normal daily activities, bacteria are often introduced into the blood stream. This can be due to such routine activities such as brushing one's teeth, chewing gum, or having a bowel movement. These bacteria enter the venous circulation and can return to the heart. Under normal circumstances, most of these bacteria are removed by macrophages in the lungs. If there is a right-to-left shunt, however, this mechanism is bypassed, and the bacteria can pass into the arterial circulation. Once there, they can be the cause of abscesses. The most serious is brain abscess, which is a known complication of congenital heart disease with right-to-left shunting.

Clots are the other source of paradoxical embolization. A small number of spontaneous thrombi can form in the venous system because of stasis resulting from sitting or remaining in one position for a long time. This risk can be increased by certain factors, such as smoking, high estrogen levels, dehydration, or hypercoagulable states. These small thrombi are normally filtered out in the lungs but can embolize to the left side if there is a right-to-left shunt.

Of course, the presence of a right-to-left shunt can also lead to significant cyanosis, which, in turn, can lead to increase in the number of red cells, resulting in an increased blood viscosity. This itself leads to an increase in the coagulability of the blood. This means that a prominent right-to-left shunt can be a risk factor for embolization in two synergistic ways.

Finally, right-to-left shunting carries special embolization risks during certain procedures. Orthopedic surgery often involves the placing of prosthetic devices or nails into the marrow of the bone. These can result in significantly elevated intramedullary pressures and embolization of fat and marrow into the venous circulation, which may then find their way to the systemic circulation. Similarly, during vaginal delivery, embolic material may find its way into the venous circulation and, in a patient with right-to-left shunt, could propagate to the systemic circulation as well.

Ductal Dependence

Not all consequences of shunts are bad for the patient. Many different combinations of defects lead to inadequate blood flow to either the pulmonary or systemic circulation. In these cases, the open ductus arteriosus at birth provides a source of "supplemental" blood flow. When the ductus closes, this additional blood flow will be lost, and the patient will become critically ill. This phenomenon is called ductal dependence. When this happens, prompt care is critical and usually consists of administering prostaglandin E_1 intravenously, which causes the ductal muscle to relax and the ductus to open again. This stabilizes the infant so that a more permanent, surgical solution can be found.

Any one of the problems discussed previously under Role of Flow in the Development of Cardiac Structures can lead to ductal dependence. For example, if there is severe pulmonic stenosis, soon after birth the ductus will allow sufficient pulmonary blood flow to allow adequate oxygenation. When the ductus closes, however, there will be too little blood flowing through the lungs. Similarly, on the left side of the heart, if there is mitral atresia, there will be sufficient blood flow to the body through the ductus to maintain circulation at first. When the ductus closes, the systemic circulation will drop quickly, resulting in shock.

Transposition of the great arteries is also a ductal-dependent abnormality. If there is no ductus, the systemic and pulmonary circulations are parallel, with no way for sys-temic blood to reach the pulmonary circulation to be oxygenated. The open ductus provides just such a pathway, until it closes. In addition to prostaglandin E_1, another alternative in this case is a balloon atrial septostomy, which is a procedure in which a catheter with a balloon attached is passed through the foramen ovale, inflated, and then withdrawn through the atrial septum, resulting in a larger opening. Because many of the surgical procedures for transposition of the great arteries require that the atrial septum be removed anyway, this does not cause a problem with later repair. However, this procedure is not performed if an arterial switch repair is planned, because the septostomy results in an atrial septal defect, which would then need to be repaired.

Examination of the Fetus

The examination of the fetus is by any criterion a special case of the echocardiographic examination. We do not have any symptoms at all, relying completely on auscultation and other indirect methods of examination for our findings. We are not able to position the patient directly and must chase our echocardiographic windows as the fetus moves. At the same time, the lungs are filled with fluid, allowing us to easily image the heart through them, so that we have more potential windows than at any other time during life. Finally, the physiology of the circulation is unique, making some defects difficult or impossible to detect, whereas other defects that are either incompatible with postnatal life or cause severe symptoms after birth can be present without causing any fetal distress.

The reasons for examination in the fetus are different as well. Most fetal cardiac examinations are part of a routine screening examination of the entire fetus. The examinations that focus on the heart are usually because there is a risk factor in the pregnancy, there is another fetal anomaly already identified, or there is a heart abnormality or arrhythmia identified in a screening examination. With the exception of the case of rhythm disturbances, the method for each of these situations is very similar.

The range and potential complexity of abnormalities detectable on a fetal cardiac examination are quite large. In general, patients with defects are probably best handled at centers with highly specialized expertise in this area as well as by teams capable of addressing the many facets of problems with which these patients present. In spite of that caveat, many centers may be called on to do more basic screening, and the thrust of this book overall is toward such centers as well as those who are just learning the ultrasound examination.

Method of Examination

Because the fetal heart is not fully formed before the end of the first trimester, there is little point in attempting an examination before then. I have performed successful examinations of the fetal heart as early as 16 weeks of gestation, but many cardiac-specific examinations are done much later for both practical as well as medical reasons. As noted later, some defects may progress or even develop later than 16 weeks as a result of abnormal flow patterns.

The mother is usually placed in the supine position on an examining bed. Late in pregnancy this position can cause discomfort or lightheadedness because of compression of the inferior vena cava by the uterus. If this is the case, the mother can be examined in the lateral decubitus position, although this does not allow as wide an echo "window."

Because the entire lower abdomen can be used as an echo "window," larger amounts of ultrasonic coupling gel are frequently used compared with other "pediatric" examinations. Many laboratories use gel warmers to lessen the discomfort associated with large amounts of cold gel applied to the abdomen. For the sonographer accustomed to newborn and premature infant examinations, the amount of pressure on the transducer that the mother can tolerate without discomfort may come as a surprise. One additional approach that is sometimes helpful early in gestation or for the obese mother is the use of a transvaginal probe.

There are at least three major differences between prenatal and postnatal examinations (Table 3–1). The fetal lungs are filled with fluid, so it is possible to image through them, increasing the available echo windows. There are no external landmarks, so all of the image orientation must be based on the images themselves. Finally, the fetus

Table 3–1. Unique Characteristics of Prenatal Ultrasound Examinations

Prenatal Difference	Consequences
Fetal lungs filled with fluid	Increased echocardiographic access, more "windows"
No external landmarks	Need to use internal, image-related landmarks
Fetus moves freely	Opportunistic, rapid examination a necessity

can move relatively freely, so the sonographer must be a persistent opportunist!

Although the survey examination in the fetus will rarely be possible in a specified sequence, its goal should include everything in the standard survey examination (Box 3–1). There are several significant points of difference from other age groups, summarized in Table 3–2. The first is that the normal fetal heart has significant shunts at both the atrial level, through the foramen ovale, and at the arterial level, through the ductus arteriosus. This means that the pressures on the right and left sides of the heart are similar, and chamber sizes are similar. The second point is that the blood flow through the lungs is markedly diminished, making the diagnosis of abnormal flow resulting from stenosis of the pulmonic valve or pulmonary arteries more difficult. These first two differences also make the utility of Doppler less in the fetus than in older age groups. Third, the range of defects possible in the fetus is larger and biased toward more severe defects than in the newborn, because some fetuses with severe defects never reach delivery, so defects incompatible with life after birth are more common. Fourth, some defects may develop during the second and third trimesters. These are defects that result from abnormal flow patterns, as discussed in Chapter 2 under Role of Blood Flow in the Development of Cardiac Structures. For this reason, findings that are absent early in the pregnancy may develop later. Finally, abnormalities of cardiac position are usually easy to detect after birth, on physical examination or x-ray film, but in the fetus the cardiac position is unknown except by the echocardiogram, so determination of cardiac position should be included early. This also assists in the orientation of views later.

To determine the position of the heart in the thorax, it is necessary to determine the overall orientation of the fetus relative to the transducer. This is usually done most easily by finding the head and obtaining a transverse view. Then the transducer is

---

BOX 3–1
ECHOCARDIOGRAPHIC SURVEY EXAMINATION IN THE FETUS

Cardiac situs
  Heart in left chest
  Apex pointed to left
Two ventricles
  Interventricular septum intact
  Equal in size
Two atria
  Equal in size
  Left atrium <1.5 times aortic diameter
  Foramen ovale open
Atrioventricular valves
  Each into respective ventricle
  Tricuspid slightly displaced toward apex
Semilunar valves
  Each from respective ventricle
  Pulmonic valve anterior
Great arteries
  Pulmonary artery and aorta cross
  Ductus arteriosus open
  Complete aortic arch visualized and patent

Table 3–2. Differences in Fetal Heart Physiology/Anatomy

Fetal Difference	Consequences
Shunts at atrial/ductal levels	Pressures/chamber sizes similar
Less blood flow through lungs	Abnormalities of pulmonic valve/artery less apparent
Severe defects more common	Range of possibilities larger
Development not complete	Some defects resulting from impaired flow may develop later
Situs uncertain	Early situs determination necessary

checked to be sure that the transverse view is in the standard orientation (i.e., from the foot of the fetus looking toward the head, and not a mirror image). This can be done by angling the transducer back and forth in the plane of the image as well as perpendicular to the plane of the image, toward the neck and top of the head, and seeing whether the motions make sense from that orientation. If it is a mirror image, the transducer must be rotated 180 degrees. Then the transducer can be angled or moved toward the foot of the fetus until the heart comes into view, and the position can be determined.

Some authors suggested that the four-chamber view is sufficient for a screening examination (Fig. 3–1). This view definitely is the easiest to obtain reliably and certainly has the most information needed for the screening examination. It does not provide information on the great vessels or their relationship, however. Sometimes it is possible to obtain a glimpse of the great vessels and their relationship by angling the plane of the transducer from the four-chamber view to obtain a nonstandard view. It is often easier, though, to just look for the standard views, which show the relationship of the great vessels, such as the long-

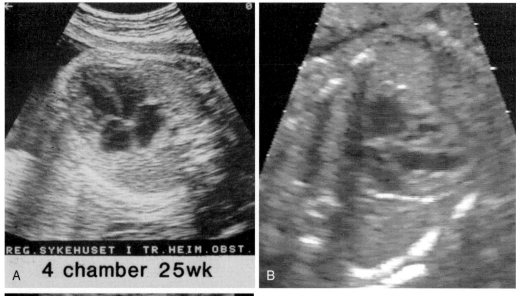

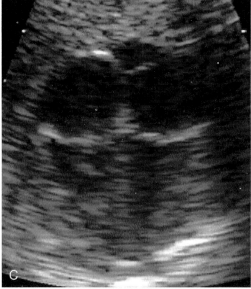

Figure 3–1. *A,* Standard four-chamber view in a normal fetus. Note that the spine can be seen to the right of the image and that the atrioventricular valve on the left is slightly displaced toward the apex relative to the other atrioventricular valve. This indicates that it is the tricuspid valve and that it is anterior. *B,* Another orientation of the same type of view in another fetus. The views are not as standardized because of the inability to position the fetus. The spine is to the lower left. The upper ventricle is the right ventricle, with the tricuspid valve slightly displaced toward the ventricular apex. *C,* Another four-chamber view, with the tricuspid valve on the left of the image. In this case, the widely open patent foramen ovale is also visible.

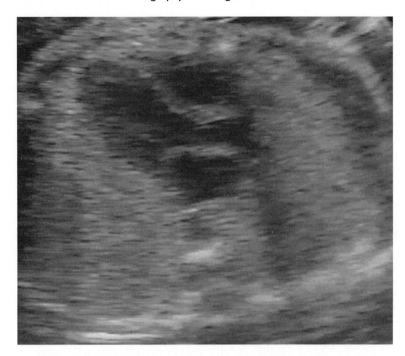

Figure 3–2. In this long-axis image of a normal fetal heart, the spine is at the bottom of the image and the right ventricle is at the top. The left atrium is close to the spine, and it is possible to see the left ventricular outflow tract and ascending aorta.

axis view (Fig. 3–2) and the short-axis view (Fig. 3–3). Using the four-chamber view alone for screening leads to only about 40% of significant, detectable lesions being found. Another view that is occasionally obtainable is that of the complete aortic arch (Fig. 3–4).

A common normal variant that is seen in the fetus but not so apparent in newborns or older children is the "golf ball" in the left ventricle (Fig. 3–5). This is caused by fibrous tissue at the tip of the papillary muscles causing a disproportionate echogenicity in the small left ventricle.

Pregnancy With High Risk of Heart Disease

A common reason for a detailed examination of the fetal heart is that there is some reason to suspect a higher incidence of heart disease than in the general population. Table 3–3 lists some of the reasons that would increase the risk of congenital heart disease in a particular pregnancy. In general, it is useful to categorize the risk factors into maternal and fetal. Maternal risk factors are those that are based on maternal disease, family history, or maternal exposure to tox-

ins, drugs, or infectious agents. Fetal risk factors are those that are detectable by examination of the fetus.

Maternal, noncardiac disease is a significant risk factor. Maternal diabetes is certainly a risk factor for a type of myocardial hypertrophy that resembles hypertrophic cardiomyopathy in appearance and physiology but differs in that it gradually resolves in the affected infants, does not have the same genetic predispositions, and is rarely obstructive. Maternal systemic lupus erythematosus is an important risk factor for congenital complete heart block. In fact, maternal lupus may sometimes be detected only after the detection of high-grade atrioventricular conduction block in the fetus or newborn.

Maternal exposure is also an important risk factor. Exposures can be categorized as medications, toxins, or infectious agents. With better education, these are becoming less common. The most common are listed in Table 3–3 and include rubella and alcohol exposure.

The contribution of congenital heart disease in the family is a more complex topic. To fully assess the risk, a careful history of at least the first-order relatives is necessary. For the fetus, this means the parents and

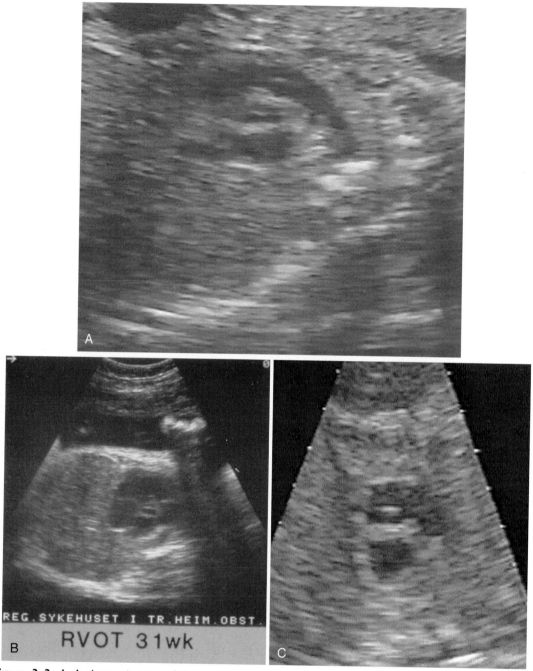

Figure 3–3. *A,* A short-axis view of the aortic valve in cross-section and the right ventricular outflow tract, pulmonic valve, and main pulmonary artery in a longitudinal section. This clearly shows that the two great vessels cross. *B,* A more standard short-axis view showing the aortic valve in cross-section, the right and left atria, the tricuspid valve, right ventricular outflow, and pulmonic valve. *C,* A short-axis view of the ventricles, demonstrating early equal size.

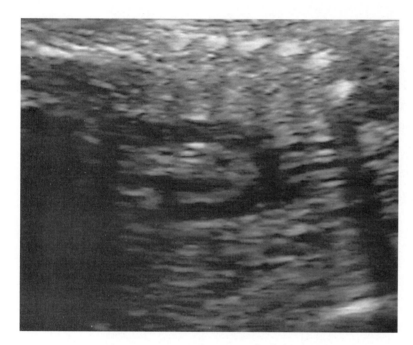

Figure 3–4. The aortic arch can sometimes be visualized in its entirety. Here, the fetus's back is at the top of the image; therefore, the descending aorta is also at the top. It is possible to see some of the arch vessels clearly on the right of the image.

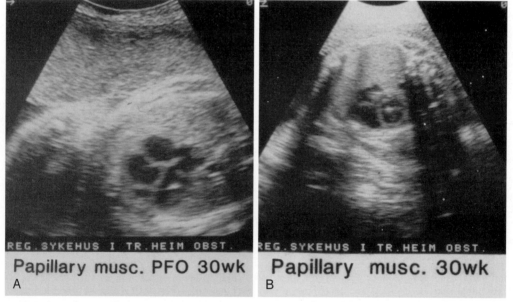

Figure 3–5. Prominent reflectivity of the tip of a papillary muscle in the left ventricle, or "golf ball," seen in the four-chamber view *(A)* and the short-axis view *(B)*.

Table 3–3. Factors Associated With Increased Risk of Fetal CHD

Factor	Most Common Congenital Heart Disease
Maternal Disease	
Diabetes	Left ventricular hypertrophy, possibly VSD, TGA
Phenylketonuria	Tetralogy of Fallot, VSD, ASD
Systemic lupus	High grade AV conduction block
Maternal Exposure	
Rubella	PDA, peripheral pulmonic stenosis, VSD, ASD
Alcohol	VSD, ASD, PDA
Lithium	Ebstein's anomaly
Hydantoin	Pulmonic stenosis, aortic stenosis
Genetic	
CHD in family	Variable, see text
Fetal	
Chromosome abnormality	Variable, depends on abnormality
Other defect noted	Variable, depends on nature of defects

ASD, atrial septal defect; AV, atrioventricular; CHD, congenital heart disease; PDA, patent ductus arteriosus; TGA, transposition of great arteries; VSD, ventricular septal defect.

siblings. The relative risk depends on the number of relatives affected, the type of defects, and even which relatives are affected. As a general rule, if the mother has congenital heart disease, the risk is increased by a greater amount than if the father has congenital heart disease, a fact that indicates that this is not simple inheritance. The degree of increase depends on the type of congenital heart disease. If one sibling has congenital heart disease, the increase in risk is usually similar to that if the father has congenital heart disease. There is considerable variability in the recurrence risk as a function of the type of defect, even among different studies of this relationship, so it is difficult to make generalizations. Finally, the number of affected relatives will affect the risk of congenital heart disease in the fetus.

Some numbers can help to illustrate this. If the mother has a ventricular septal defect, the risk for the fetus is 6% to 10% for having congenital heart disease. If the

father has a ventricular septal defect, however, the risk is only 2%. If one sibling has a ventricular septal defect, the risk is 3%; if two siblings have ventricular septal defects, the risk is 10%. For tetralogy of Fallot, the numbers are as follows: mother, 2.5%; father, 1.5%; one sibling, 2.5%; two siblings, 8%. For aortic stenosis, the respective risks are as follows: mother, 13% to 18%; father, 3%; one sibling, 2%; two siblings, 6%.

It is important to note that the recurrence risk is not exclusively for the same type of defect. Although there is a mild tendency to have recurrence of the same type of defect, there is an overall increase in all types of defects. Even though this is true, the parents are most likely concerned about recurrence of the particular defect or defects present in the family, and reassuring them about the absence of those defects is important if this is possible based on the examination.

Maternal congenital heart disease can also affect fetal development and survival because of effects on the maternal circulation and oxygen saturation, even without causing heart defects in the fetus. This is discussed in Chapter 6 under Assessing Risk of Pregnancy in the Patient with Congenital Heart Disease.

The fetal factors are primarily based on chromosomal abnormalities or abnormalities detectable on the ultrasound examination. The presence of a chromosomal abnormality increases the risk of a cardiac defect, generally to more than 30%. The actual frequency and type of defect depends on the exact chromosomal abnormality, but the most common are discussed later.

The presence of any noncardiac structural congenital defect detected on examination will increase the chance of finding a cardiac defect. This is because many cardiac anomalies are part of syndromes, and a large percentage of all anomalies are not isolated. Finally, growth abnormalities and hydrops can be caused by cardiac anomalies or failure and, therefore, warrant a detailed cardiac examination.

Diagnosis of Abnormality

The diagnosis of defects in the fetus is somewhat different than in other age groups because it is usually completely based on the echocardiographic examination, with no presenting symptoms or clinical signs. This means that the range of possible diagnoses cannot be limited by the presentation and, therefore, must be larger than in other age groups. Combining this with the fact that lesions that are uniformly fatal can also be found creates a range of lesions that is actually much larger than for any other age group. For this reason, it is helpful to approach the screening examination as an "inventory" of features that are either present or absent and then synthesize these findings into a diagnosis or syndrome. This is similar to the approach suggested by one of my professors in hematology in medical school, Dr. Paul Kreger, who believed that we should first take the "German" approach, systematically describing our findings, and then we should take the "French" approach, philosophizing about what it all means.

The screening examination as outlined here is also similar to the segmental approach used in many textbooks of congenital heart disease. In particular, we start by identifying the cardiac and visceral organ situs. Subsequent identification is along the flow patterns of blood. We then identify the venous connections, followed by atrial anatomy, atrioventricular connections, ventricles, ventriculoarterial connections, and great artery anatomy. Again, because of the opportunistic character of the fetal examination, this approach is how we organize the information obtained after the examination rather than a sequence of acquisition!

Even if all of these features are identified and are normal, we cannot be certain that there is no congenital heart disease. Because of the differences between prenatal and postnatal physiology, many smaller lesions are difficult or impossible to detect prenatally. Only about 30% of congenital heart defects are severe enough to cause problems immediately after birth, but fortunately these also usually cause structural abnormalities of sufficient severity to be detectable on a fetal ultrasound examination. A detailed, cardiac-specific examination should detect virtually all of these.

Once we have our inventory, even if incomplete, we can start to use our knowledge of the patterns of malformation to look for possible associated problems (see Syndromes in Chapter 2). In particular, the three "embryological principles" are very helpful as a mnemonic aid to which abnormalities are likely to be associated.

Examples of Structural Defects

As noted, even though the range of possible defects in the fetus is larger than at any other age, not all defects can be diagnosed, because of the limitations imposed by physiology and resolution. In general, severe defects should be detectable, whereas the more common, lesser defects will go undetected (Box 3–2).

Following are some examples and comments on some of the detectable defects (Table 3–4).

Transposition of the Great Arteries

Transposition of the great arteries is one of the defects that cannot be detected on the

---

BOX 3–2
DETECTABILITY OF DEFECTS

Likely to be detected
  Tetralogy of Fallot
  Atrioventricular septal defect
  Truncus arteriosus
  Transposition of the great arteries
  Pulmonary atresia
  Hypoplastic left heart
  Mitral or tricuspid atresia
Less likely to be detected
  Aortic/pulmonic stenosis
  Aortic coarctation
Unlikely to be detected
  Secundum atrial septal defect
  Perimembranous ventricular septal defect

Table 3–4. Identifying Features of Particular Diagnoses

Diagnosis	View	Feature
Transposition of the great arteries	Outflow	Parallel great arteries Anterior → arch, posterior → lungs
Tetralogy of Fallot	Outflow	Malalignment VSD Overriding aorta Small main pulmonary artery
AV septal defect	Four chamber	AV valves at same level Straddling valve Inlet ventricular septal defect Primum atrial septal defect
	Short axis	Cleft mitral valve
Truncus arteriosus	Outflow	Absent pulmonary artery from ventricles Malalignment VSD Pulmonary artery from trunk
Tricuspid atresia	Four chamber	Absent tricuspid valve Ventricular septal defect Small RV

VSD, ventricular septal defect; AV, atrioventricular; RV, right ventricle.

routine four-chamber examination. This is because all four chambers appear normal, as do the cardiac septa. The key to diagnosing transposition is to identify the great arteries and their connections. Normally, the

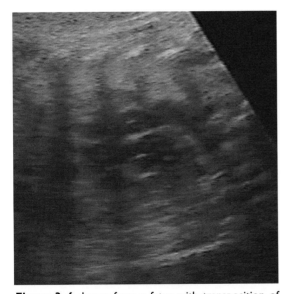

Figure 3–6. Image from a fetus with transposition of the great arteries. The two great arteries and their associated valves are visible in the same plane, which is abnormal. The aortic valve is on the top, which is anterior in the fetus, and courses to the right toward the aortic arch. The larger pulmonic valve is seen just below. The aortic valve should be posterior to the pulmonic valve.

pulmonary artery heads posteriorly shortly after its origin, whereas the aorta courses cephalad (toward the head) for a longer distance before it reaches the aortic arch. When they originate in the normal ventricles, the result is that they cross. When they are transposed, the course is parallel (Fig. 3–6). It is important to also look for additional defects such as large ventricular septal defects or pulmonic stenosis, among others, which will markedly alter the prognosis and surgical options.

Tetralogy of Fallot

Tetralogy of Fallot is also difficult to detect on the four-chamber view. This is because the normal right and left ventricular wall thicknesses are equal, so the presence of a large ventricular septal defect will not change the sizes or thickness of the ventricles. The outflow and great arteries are also not seen in the four-chamber view.

The key to the diagnosis is the overriding of the aorta, the malalignment ventricular septal defect (Fig. 3–7), and presence of a small pulmonary artery coming from the right ventricle. This distinguishes it from truncus arteriosus, in which the pulmonary artery does not arise from the ventricles at all.

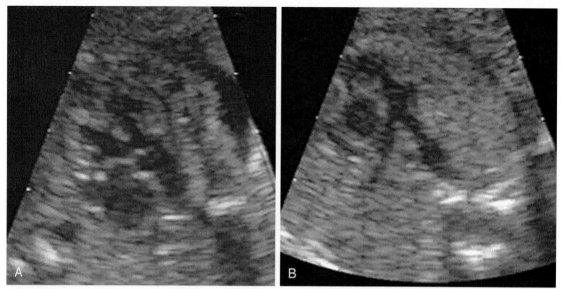

Figure 3–7. A, The aorta overrides the ventricular septum in a fetus with tetralogy of Fallot. The ascending aorta is directed downward and to the right. B, This image from the same fetus shows the main pulmonary artery and its branches, which are hypoplastic in comparison to the aorta, seen in cross-section to their left. Note that this defect would be difficult or impossible to detect from a standard four-chamber view.

Atrioventricular Septal Defect

In atrioventricular septal defects, the four-chamber view is always abnormal. At the very least, the portions of the atrioventricular valves that are visible will appear to be at the same level, which is distinctly abnormal. In some cases, the atrial defect and ventricular defect will be easily visible, and there will appear to be a single straddling valve (Fig. 3–8).

Truncus Arteriosus

In truncus arteriosus there is always a large ventricular septal defect of the malalignment variety, and the trunk is overriding the ventricular septum. In this sense, it is similar to tetralogy of Fallot. The difference is that it is often possible to identify the pulmonary arteries and their method of connection to the trunk, and there is no pulmonary artery originating in the ventricles (Fig. 3–9). If there is a main pulmonary artery arising from the trunk, which then branches, this is called type I. If there is no main pulmonary artery but the two branches have a common origin from the trunk, it is called type II. If the two pulmonary arteries have completely separate origins, this is called type III. If there are no pulmonary artery branches, this is called pulmonary atresia, although it used to be

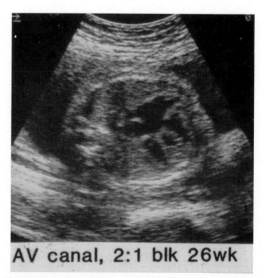

AV canal, 2:1 blk 26wk

Figure 3–8. This four-chamber view is from a fetus with a complete atrioventricular septal defect. The spine of the fetus is to the left of the image, and the apex of the heart is pointed toward the lower right. Note that there appears to be a single atrioventricular valve straddling the ventricular septum. Also there is a clear defect in the interatrial septum in the portion near the valve; the septal remnant is seen as a small ridge at the upper left of the atrial wall.

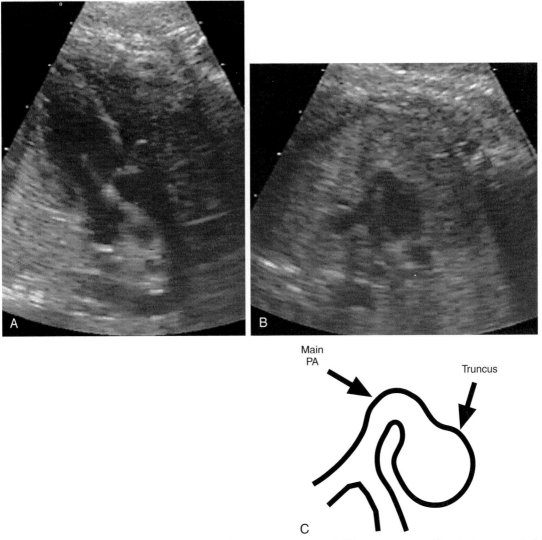

Figure 3–9. These images are from a fetus with truncus arteriosus. A, The truncus overrides the interventricular septum in a long-axis view. B, A short-axis view of the truncus, with the main pulmonary artery coming off anteriorly and then coursing posteriorly before it branches. This indicates that this is a type I truncus arteriosus because there is a main pulmonary artery. C, A line drawing of the structures in B.

called type IV truncus. This grading of type correlates to a degree with the degree of difficulty with a surgical repair.

Tricuspid Atresia

In tricuspid atresia, the four-chamber view will be markedly abnormal. As expected, there is no functioning tricuspid valve, and in its place there is either a muscular ridge or an imperforate membrane. The right ventricle is usually small, and there is a large ventricular septal defect

permitting flow to the right ventricular outflow tract and pulmonary artery. It is important to verify the presence, location, and size of the great vessels because this can have a significant influence on therapeutic options.

PARTICULAR SYNDROMES

In addition to the defects noted previously, which either are isolated or involve very typical combinations, there are a number of fairly common syndromes. In some cases these are genetic, with known chromosomal abnormalities. Others are combinations of defects that have a wide variability of expression (Table 3–5).

Down Syndrome (Trisomy 21)

The incidence of cardiac defects in patients with Down syndrome is approximately 50%. Although all types of cardiac defects can occur, there is an excess of defects of the endocardial cushion type, especially atrioventricular septal defects, so that this is commonly thought of in association with Down syndrome. In spite of this, the range of defects occurring in Down syndrome is very wide and encompasses the entire range of defects.

Trisomy 18

This very serious chromosomal defect is primarily associated with ventricular septal defects and patent ductus arteriosus, although others may occur.

Turner's Syndrome (XO Syndrome)

The fetus with Turner's syndrome is usually identified by features other than the cardiac defects, including nuchal cystic hygroma and generalized edema. A wide range of cardiac defects have been associated with Turner's syndrome, but the most common is coarctation of the aorta.

Hypoplastic Left Heart

As mentioned in Chapter 2, any isolated defect that results in a decreased flow to left-sided structures will result in hypoplasia of the "downstream" structures as well. Although mitral hypoplasia and atresia and left ventricular hypoplasia or atresia are usually present, the critical element that must be present is aortic valve and ascending aortic hypoplasia or atresia (Fig. 3–10). This is because some variants include ventricular septal defect, which results in flow to the left ventricle and a "normal" size, although the hypoplastic aortic valve and ascending aorta are more important in determining the overall prognosis and management. The crucial question is whether there will be adequate flow to the ascending aorta once the ductus has closed after birth.

This cannot be reliably detected on a four-chamber view because the aorta is not seen. We must look at the aortic outflow, at the very least. Norms for ascending aortic size versus gestational age have been developed. In general, the growth of the aortic

Table 3–5. Possible Features of Particular Syndromes

Diagnosis	View	Feature
Down syndrome (trisomy 21)	Four chamber	Atrioventricular septal defect
	Various	Other defects
Trisomy 18	Outflow	Ventricular septal defect
		Pulmonic stenosis
Turner's syndrome (XO)	Aortic arch	Coarctation of the aorta
	Outflow	Aortic stenosis
	Four chamber	Atrial septal defect
Hypoplastic left heart	Four chamber	Small left ventricle
		Mitral atresia
	Outflow	Small aorta
Premature closure of foramen ovale	Four chamber	Large right heart
		Small foramen ovale
		Pleural effusions

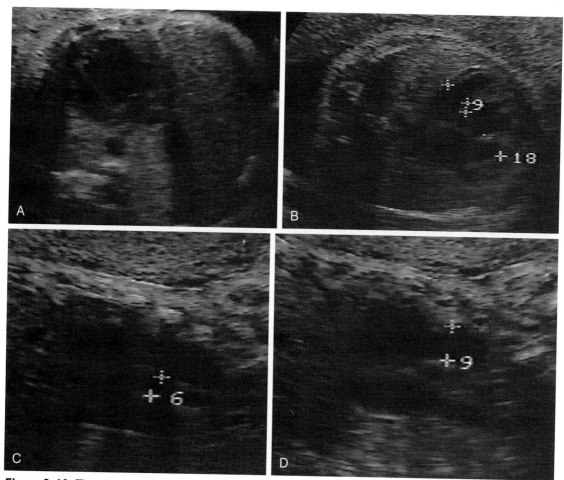

Figure 3–10. These images are from a fetus with hypoplastic left-sided heart. *A,* A view between a short axis and four chamber; the spine of the fetus is at the lower left. The enlarged right ventricle is at the top of the image, and there is a slit-like left ventricle to its left. *B,* The relative dimensions of the right and left ventricles at end-diastole; the right ventricle measures twice the size of the left. *C,* Measurement of the ascending aorta, which is hypoplastic. *D,* The larger pulmonary artery.

root is linear, and by 28 weeks the diameter should be greater than 5 mm, and by about 36 weeks the diameter should be greater than 7 mm.

Premature Closure of Foramen Ovale

This syndrome is characterized by enlargement of the right ventricle, pleural effusions, and narrowing or closure of the foramen ovale. The key to diagnosis is the absence of other defects. The infants often have respiratory problems after birth, which can persist. The cause of this syndrome is unclear. The name of the syndrome

indicates the leading hypothesis as to the cause of the syndrome, although, to me, the description seems inadequate. It seems more likely that the syndrome is caused by inappropriately low pulmonary vascular resistance, leading to increased pulmonary flow, which in turn leads to increased left atrial filling and closure of the foramen ovale as well as pleural effusions.

Arrhythmia

The normal way of diagnosing rhythm disturbances in other age groups is through the electrocardiogram. Although it is possible to perform an electrocardiogram on a fetus using special techniques, it is usually easier and more convenient to obtain the same information from the echocardiographic examination.

Ventricular activity is easy to record using M-mode. We can see the ventricular contractions and record any irregularity. If we can find a beam direction that includes both of the ventricles and an atrium, we can usually see the atrial contractions and relate these to the ventricular contractions (Fig. 3–11). If we are unable to find a beam direction that allows us to record both of these levels of activity, it is virtually always possible to record the atrioventricular valve motion on the same M-mode recording as the ventricular activity, allowing us to see the results of atrial contraction as the mitral or tricuspid A wave (Fig. 3–12).

As always, the essentials of arrhythmia diagnosis are to determine the atrial and ventricular rates, the relationship of the two, and any irregularities. With this information in hand, we can make a useful diagnosis of the rate, rhythm, and any disorders.

The range of common rhythm distur-

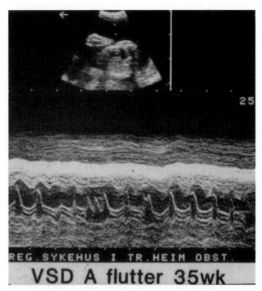

Figure 3–12. M-mode through an atrioventricular valve of a 35-week fetus with atrial flutter and variable atrioventricular block. Note that the flutter waves are visible when the conduction is blocked briefly.

bances in the fetus is somewhat smaller than in older age groups. For convenience, we can divide the rhythm disturbances into slow rhythms, rapid rhythms, and irregular rhythms (Table 3–6). The normal fetus has a heart rate that is quite high and varies throughout the pregnancy. For simplicity, we can define the rule-of-thumb limits of 100 beats per minute as the lower limit of normal and 160 beats per minute as the upper limit of normal.

Constant bradycardia, or an abnormally slow heart rate, is rare in the fetus. When it is present, it is frequently a sign of a serious abnormality. Variable bradycardia, however, is common, especially during labor. In that case, slowing of the heart rate, or "deceleration," occurs during the contractions. So-called late decelerations occurring after contractions are a sign of fetal distress.

The two types of constant bradycardia that are most common are sinus bradycardia (in which there is normal atrioventricular conduction, the atria are beating at a slow rate, and the ventricles are beating at the same rate) and heart block (in which the atria are beating at one rate and the ventricles are beating at a slower rate).

Sinus bradycardia almost always indi-

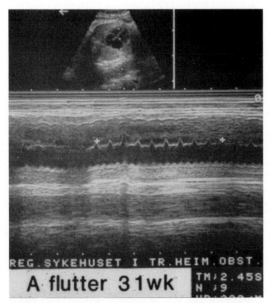

Figure 3–11. This is an M-mode with the ventricle on top and atrium on the bottom of a 31-week fetus with atrial flutter with 2:1 block and a ventricular rate of 220. It is possible to see the flutter waves in the atrium below and the atrioventricular valves opening every other flutter wave.

Table 3–6. Fetal Rhythm Disorders

Type	Diagnoses	Associations
Bradycardia	Late decelerations Sinus bradycardia Heart block	Fetal distress Fetal distress Conduction abnormality (SLE) Ventricular inversion Atrioventricular septal defect Single ventricle Other complex defects
Tachycardia	Atrial tachycardia Atrial flutter	Failure, hydrops Failure, hydrops
Irregular rhythm	Premature atrial beats Sinus pause Premature ventricular beats	Normal, rare atrial tachycardia Normal early in pregnancy Normal, less frequent

SLE, systemic lupus erythematosus.

cates a significant, noncardiac abnormality. Heart block, however, is always cardiac in origin. In more than two-thirds of fetuses with complete heart block it is the only abnormality; for example, it is frequent in fetuses of mothers with systemic lupus erythematosus. In about one-third of fetuses with heart block, it is the result of a severe structural heart disease, such as ventricular inversion, left atrial isomerism, complete atrioventricular septal defect, or single ventricle (Box 3–3).

On echocardiographic examination, the ventricular rate is quite slow, often in the 50 to 60 beat per minute range (Fig. 3–13). The atrial and ventricular contractions may have a fixed relationship, such as two atrial beats to each ventricular beat. In this case the fetus has second-degree atrioventricular block with 2:1 atrioventicular conduction. If there is no relationship between the atrial and ventricular contractions, the rhythm is said to be third-degree heart block. In that case, the chance of having an associated structural defect is quite high, probably at least 50%. Even when there is no structural heart disease, these fetuses are at risk for heart failure, which presents in the fetus as hydrops (Fig. 3–14). For this reason, a detailed examination is particularly important. See Box 3–4 for the sufficient screening examination.

Tachycardia in the fetus is more common than constant bradycardia. If it is due to a rhythm disturbance rather than a physiological response, the rate is usually quite high, typically greater than 220 beats per minute. Identification of the relationship between atrial and ventricular contractions is key to an accurate diagnosis; the most common rhythm disturbances are supraventricular tachycardia and atrial flutter. The former has 1:1 conduction from the atrium to the ventricle (Fig. 3–15), whereas the latter has variable (1:2 or 1:3) conduction (see Figs. 3–11 and 3–12). There is no significant

---

BOX 3–3
POTENTIAL ABNORMAL FINDINGS IN COMPLETE HEART BLOCK

Cardiac situs
  Situs inversus or ambiguous
Ventricles
  Ventricular inversion
  Large ventricular septal defect
  Atrioventricular septal defect
Atria
  Large primum atrial septal defect
  Single atrium
Atrioventricular valves
  Straddling valve
  Two valves into one ventricle (double-inlet left ventricle or double-inlet right ventricle)
Semilunar valves
  Malalignment defects
Great arteries
  Transposition

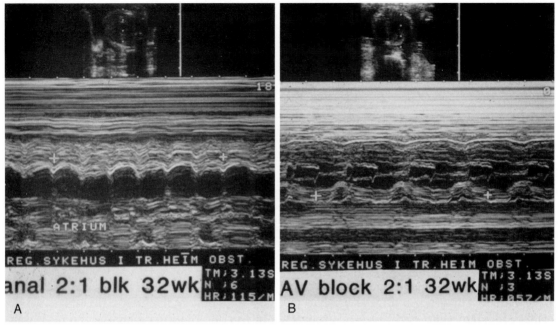

Figure 3–13. *A,* The atrial M-mode from a 32-week fetus with 2:1 atrioventricular block. The rate is 115, which is normal. *B,* The atrioventricular valves on the same patient, with a rate of 57.

increase in structural heart disease in patients with either of these rhythm disturbances. In spite of this, both rhythm disturbances can lead to hydrops and fetal distress or even death. For this reason, it is important to assess the overall function as well as diagnose the rhythm.

Particular features to look for are increased ventricular size and decreased function, pericardial and pleural effusions, and edema and ascites (hydrops). Fetuses with these findings often also show decreased activity. Any of these findings can be indicators of poorly tolerated tachyarrhythmia and indications for treatment (see Fig. 3–14).

The final category is an irregular heartbeat. In most cases these are extra beats and are normal variants. Most extra beats are premature supraventricular beats.

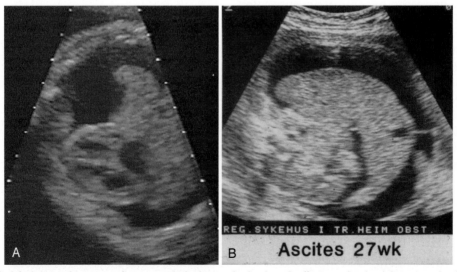

Figure 3–14. Images from two fetuses with hydrops. *A,* A pleural effusion, clearly delineating the heart and collapsed lung. *B,* Ascites surrounding the liver.

These can be diagnosed echocardiographically by the premature atrial contraction followed by a ventricular contraction or, if the atrial beat is blocked, a pause in ventricular activity (Fig. 3–16). These are quite common in normal fetuses and are of virtually no significance. Rarely, frequent premature supraventricular beats can lead to a supraventricular tachycardia or atrial flutter. There is no significant increase in structural heart disease in fetuses with premature supraventricular beats.

One common normal variant bears comment in this context. Early in the second trimester, immaturity of the sinoatrial node can lead to alarming sinus pauses, but this is a normal variant.

EFFECTS ON THE HEART OF OTHER DISEASE

Many fetal disorders can adversely effect the heart. These are primarily through volume loading or a direct toxic effect on the heart. As would be expected, volume loading, whatever the cause, results in increased chamber size with hyperdynamic function. An example of volume overload is anemia resulting from Rh incompatibility. A heart adversely affected by toxins will also be dilated but will have decreased contractility. This is usually due to sepsis.

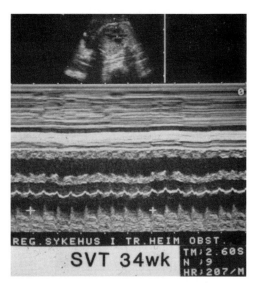

Figure 3–15. This M-mode shows the right ventricle on the top and the left atrium on the bottom. There is a one-to-one correspondence between the beats, but the overall rate is high, at 207 beats per minute, so this is supraventricular tachycardia.

> **BOX 3–4**
> **SUFFICIENT EXAMINATION IN HEART BLOCK**
>
> Cardiac situs
>   Heart in left chest
>   Apex pointed to left
> Two ventricles
>   Interventricular septum intact
>   Equal in size
> Two atria
>   Atrial septum intact
> Atrioventricular valves
>   Each into respective ventricle
>   Tricuspid slightly displaced toward apex
> Semilunar valves
>   Each from respective ventricle
>   Pulmonic valve anterior
> Great arteries
>   Pulmonary artery and aorta cross

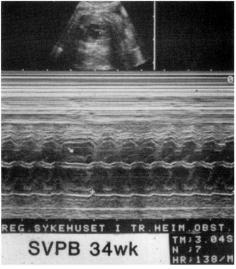

Figure 3–16. M-mode from a 34-week fetus with a supraventricular premature beat. The rhythm is regular until there is a long pause, resulting from the blocked premature atrial beat.

Chapter 4

Examination of the Newborn and Infant

The examination of the newborn can be considered either more difficult or easier than the examination in other age groups depending on one's perspective. It is more difficult because there is little clinical history to guide us, and the range of possible defects to be detected is large. It is easier because the echocardiographic windows of the newborn are usually quite adequate to allow imaging of all structures, and the newborn and infant are not afraid of the examination.

Because of this, an examination that rules out a cardiac cause of the problem can be quite rapid in the newborn. If an abnormality is found, however, the range of possibilities is so large that it may take a while to determine all of the details.

METHOD OF EXAMINATION

Infants are actually quite simple to understand. Their needs are limited: food, warmth, elimination, and human contact. Satisfying these needs is key to their health and growth, and to a successful examination.

For this reason it is often most expedient to examine the infant wherever he or she normally would be. This is mandatory in premature infants, who need to be kept warm in warming beds or isolettes, but it is also desirable for larger infants who are warm and comfortable in their cribs and blankets. The marginal benefit gained by placing an infant on an examining table is often lost when the infant becomes fussy because of the position. Larger, term infants can be placed on an examining table if they are wrapped in blankets to keep them warm, only exposing the chest for the examination.

The problem of examining infants in the neonatal intensive care unit bears some comment. There are many challenges because there is little space between the beds and often much equipment such as ventilators at the head of the bed. The newborn may be in an isolette with small "portholes" for access, further limiting positioning of the ultrasound machine. In these situations, it can be useful to learn to scan with either hand in order to be able to place the ultrasound machine on either the right or left of the patient. It may even be necessary to put the ultrasound equipment at the foot of the bed and scan upside-down, facing the feet of the patient in some cases because of equipment positioning.

Infants are quieter after they have been fed. The disadvantage to examination after feeding is that the subcostal views can be more difficult because of abdominal distension. During feeding, the infant is often more active than otherwise, and this motion can make examination difficult. If possible, it is helpful to arrange to have the infant fed a short time before the examination. If the infant has not been fed, the examination can be attempted. If fussy, the infant should be fed. Depending on the time pressure and importance of the subcostal views, these can be attempted during feeding. After feeding, all views other than the subcostal are usually much easier. Using these strategies, I have not needed to use sedation to examine any infant.

All of the standard views can be obtained in the infant, including subcostal, apical, and suprasternal. It is often easier to obtain a multitude of views, because the ribs are not as ossified as in older children, and it is possible to image through cartilage. Because of their small size, it is possible to use higher transducer frequencies. A frequency of 5 MHz is routine for term newborns and infants, whereas premature infants can often be successfully examined with higher frequencies, with resulting higher resolution. I have used frequencies up to 7.5 MHz, although this limit is probably more related to equipment design issues than to the limits of what is useful.

The echocardiographic survey examination for the newborn and infant is influenced by the transition from fetal to newborn life (Box 4–1). The right and left sides of the heart are subjected to equal pressures in the fetal period; therefore, the right and left ventricles are more equal in size and thickness than later in life (Fig. 4–1). The pulmonary vascular resistance is high at birth but falls rapidly. Right ventricular pressure is equal to systemic pressure at birth (typically about 90 mm Hg systolic for a term newborn or 70 mm Hg for a premature infant). There are normal shunts at the atrial and arterial levels (foramen ovale and ductus arteriosus) at birth, which normally become insignificant by less than 1 week of age. Thus, the normal newborn examination can change rapidly soon after birth, and knowing the age of the patient is very important to interpretation of the findings.

RESPIRATORY DISTRESS AND CONGESTIVE FAILURE

Respiratory failure must be distinguished from cardiac causes of cyanosis, which are discussed later. As a general rule, cyanosis without respiratory distress is most likely cardiac in origin, and respiratory distress in the newborn is usually not cardiac. In spite of this, there are cardiac causes for respiratory distress, and cardiac causes can complicate primary respiratory problems. When cardiac disease is accompanied by respiratory distress, it is due to congestive heart failure.

Congestive heart failure is a chronic condition characterized by high filling pressures of the left or right side of the heart and can occur in two widely different situations. The first is when there is a low cardiac output, usually as a result of obstruc-

---

BOX 4–1
ECHOCARDIOGRAPHIC SURVEY EXAMINATION IN THE NEWBORN

Two ventricles
  Interventricular septum intact
  Equal in size
Two atria
  Foramen ovale open
  Equal in size
  Left atrium <1.5 times aortic diameter
Atrioventricular valves
  Each into respective ventricle
  Tricuspid slightly displaced toward apex
  Mild to moderate tricuspid insufficiency common
Semilunar valves
  Each from respective ventricle
  Pulmonic valve anterior
  Mild pulmonic insufficiency normal
Great arteries
  Pulmonary artery and aorta cross
  Ductus arteriosus open for up to 72 h with left-to-right shunt
  No flow acceleration as a result of coarctation or peripheral pulmonic stenosis
  Mild acceleration at pulmonary artery branches normal (especially left branch)
Right ventricular pressure estimate
  Right ventricular pressure equals systemic pressure at birth
  Decreases to high 20s by 1 week

---

tion or myocardial disease. This type of failure is sometimes called "backward failure" because it is characterized by increased venous pressure ("backing up") and an inadequate cardiac output and is typically associated with hypodynamic ventricular function. For this reason, it is better referred to as hypodynamic failure. This type is less common in the newborn than the second type of heart failure, which is associated with a very high cardiac output and is caused by shunts, valvular regurgitation, or

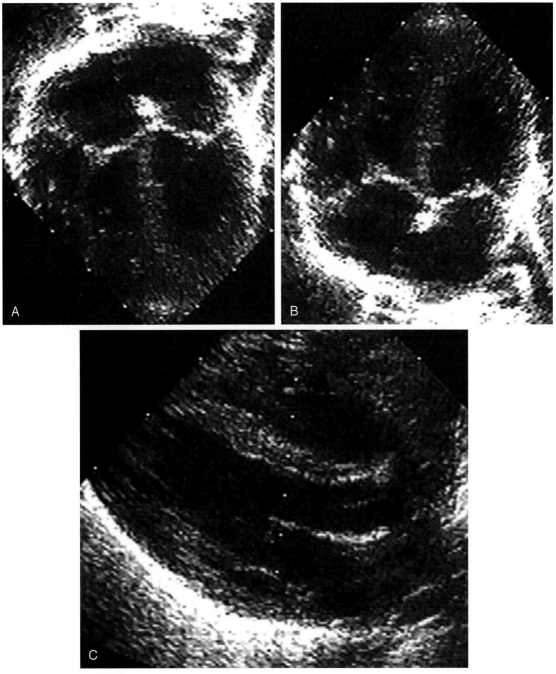

Figure 4–1. The normal newborn heart has a right ventricle that is similar in size to the left ventricle and relatively hypertrophic. This is seen in the standard pediatric *(A)* and adult *(B)* apical four-chamber views. Note also the slight offset between the tricuspid and mitral valves. *C,* The parasternal long-axis view in the same newborn.

peripheral vasodilation. This type is sometimes called "forward failure" because it has a high forward cardiac output. It is usually associated with hyperdynamic ventricular function and is, therefore, better called hyperdynamic failure.

Congestive heart failure in the infant is characterized by tachycardia, tachypnea, and poor feeding. The latter is due to difficulty breathing while feeding. The greatest exertion for the infant is feeding. Just as an older patient with congestive heart failure will have symptoms of shortness of breath during exertion, the infant can have increased respiratory rate and sweating and ultimately must stop feeding. In more advanced cases, the respiratory distress is present even when not feeding.

For respiratory distress and heart failure, the treatment is critically dependent on the precise diagnosis, and echocardiography can play a very important role in the anatomic and physiological characterization of the problem.

Pulmonary Versus Cardiac Disease

Respiratory distress is caused in part by stimulation of receptors in the lungs, and this is most commonly due to accumulation of fluid. The most common reason for a fluid build-up in the lungs of a newborn infant is respiratory distress syndrome (RDS). This is due to incomplete maturation of the lungs, with resulting incomplete inflation and fluid build-up. Infants affected by this disorder show the typical signs of respiratory distress: flaring of the nostrils, costal retractions, and grunting respiration. In mild cases, infants only need a slight oxygen supplement, whereas in more severe forms they may need mechanical ventilation. In these more severe cases, there may be additional chronic changes to the lungs called bronchopulmonary dysplasia.

Although these disorders are not caused by cardiac defects, there are cardiac consequences. The first is that there is often reflex vasoconstriction of the pulmonary vascular bed, which causes pulmonary hypertension. This can be assessed echocardiographically using the estimated right-sided pressures from tricuspid insufficiency and pulmonary insufficiency (Fig. 4–2). The second effect is that the lowered oxygen saturation can inhibit the natural closure of the ductus arteriosus. If the pulmonary pressure is lower than the systemic pressure, this will lead to a left-to-right shunt and potentially left-sided failure, with even more fluid build-up in the lungs. If the right-sided pressure is higher, it may lead to right-to-left shunting and cyanosis. The issue of evaluation of an open ductus arteriosus is discussed in detail later.

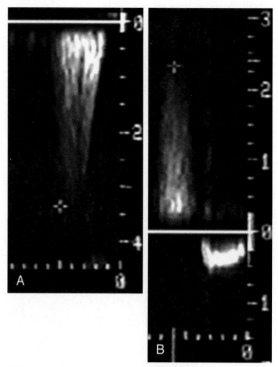

Figure 4–2. A, Tricuspid insufficiency in a 6-day-old premature infant with lung disease. The peak velocity, which is hard to see in reproduction but is marked by the cursor, is 3.3 m/s, or equivalent to a gradient of 44 mm Hg. B, The pulmonic insufficiency velocity is 2.3 m/s, which is equivalent to a gradient of 21 mm Hg.

An important clinical point is that infants with respiratory distress from lung disease may respond clinically to diuretics, even though they have no signs of heart failure on echocardiographic examination. This is because they do have an imbalance in the balance of fluid within the lungs but not because of excessive venous pressure, as is always the case with cardiac causes of respiratory distress. Rather, they have difficulty tolerating normal pulmonary venous pressure. If the chamber sizes are normal and ventricular function is normal, the heart is not the cause of the respiratory distress in spite of a response to diuretics.

Cardiac Causes of Respiratory Distress

For the heart to be the source of the respiratory distress, there must be cardiac failure with consequent build-up of fluid in the lungs. As mentioned, congestive failure can occur in two ways: volume overload (hyperdynamic failure) or pump failure with a decreased forward output (hypodynamic failure). Box 4–2 lists the various types of cardiac causes of respiratory distress.

In the case of volume overload, we should expect to be able to identify the cause and the consequences. Because we are investigating a possible cause for fluid build-up in the lungs, the volume overload would be left sided and, therefore, would be limited to ventricular septal shunts, arterial shunts, arteriovenous malformations, and either mitral or aortic regurgitation. In any case, the consequences are easiest to identify, because if

---

BOX 4–2
CARDIAC FAILURE CAUSING
RESPIRATORY DISTRESS

Volume overload
  Ventricular septal defect
  Patent ductus arteriosus
  Arteriopulmonary window
  Mitral insufficiency
  Aortic insufficiency
  (Arteriovenous malformation)
Decreased function
  Myocardial disorders
    Endocardial fibroelastosis
    Myocarditis
    Myocardial ischemia
  Rhythm disturbances
    Bradycardia
    Tachycardia
  Outflow obstruction
    Aortic stenosis
    Coarctation
  Inflow obstruction
    Mitral stenosis
    Cor triatriatum
    Anomalous pulmonary veins
  Filling disorder
    Pericardial tamponade
    Restrictive myopathy

BOX 4–3
POTENTIAL FINDINGS ON
EXAMINATION FOR CARDIAC
CAUSE OF RESPIRATORY DISTRESS

Ventricles
  Dilated left ventricle
  Thickened left ventricle (restrictive)
  Nonrestrictive ventricular septal defect
Atria
  Dilated left atrium
  "Extra" left atrial chamber (cor triatriatum)
  "Disturbed" pulmonary venous flow
Atrioventricular valves
  Severe mitral regurgitation
  Mitral stenosis
Semilunar valves
  Aortic stenosis
  Aortic regurgitation
Great arteries
  Patent ductus arteriosus
  Coarctation of the aorta
Right ventricular pressure estimate
  Normal or slight increase
Other
  Pericardial effusion
  Severe bradycardia
  Severe tachycardia
  Arteriovenous malformation

---

we have a significant source of failure, we should have chamber dilation involving either the left atrium, left ventricle, or both. Box 4–3 lists the potential findings in the echocardiographic survey examination.

A rough rule of thumb for the left atrial size is to compare it with the aortic diameter. If the diameter of the atrium is less than 1.5 times the diameter of the aorta, this is within normal limits (Fig. 4–3; see also color figure). This adjusts for the changes with growth but does not account for the differences in left atrial configuration that may occur. Sometimes the left atrium can be flattened and enlarged, somewhat like a thick pancake.

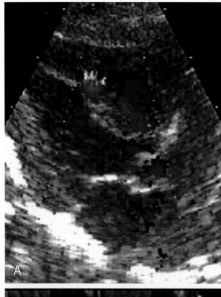

Figure 4–3. *A* (see also color figure), A parasternal long-axis view of the color flow through a small to moderate muscular ventricular septal defect in a 5-day-old newborn. *B*, The continuous-wave Doppler of the flow across the ventricular septal defect. The peak velocity is 2.8 m/s, indicating a pressure gradient of 31 mm Hg. This indicates that the right ventricular pressures are still elevated. *C*, The M-mode of the left atrial size, which is 1.7 times the size of the aorta, indicating some mild volume overload. The left ventricle is normal in size.

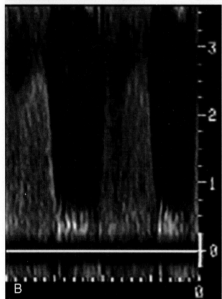

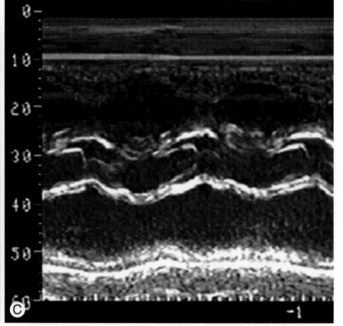

In this case, the diameter as measured by M-mode will be normal, even though the atrium is enlarged on the two-dimensional image.

Left ventricular enlargement is usually a later finding than left atrial enlargement. There are published norms of left ventricular size, but it is usually sufficient to note the shape of the ventricle and the size relative to the right ventricle (Fig. 4–4). Normally, the left ventricle has a "bullet" shape, but with volume overload the shape becomes more globular. Similarly, the normal size in the newborn is similar to the right ventricle, whereas with volume overload it becomes larger.

Once we have identified that there is failure based on enlargement of the left atrium or left ventricle or both, we should look for a shunt of the types mentioned previously. Because there are consequences of the shunt (chamber enlargement), there is significant shunt flow and the defect may not be restrictive, which in turn means that the velocity will probably be low (Fig. 4–5; see also color figure). A low-velocity shunt can be more difficult to detect than a high-velocity shunt, hence the importance of looking for the consequences first. If we see the consequences, we are going to look harder for the cause.

If valvular regurgitation is the cause, it should be easier to detect because even massive insufficiency still allows significant pressure gradients on the systemic side of the heart. Similarly, the distinction between a primary myocardial disease and volume overload caused by a shunt is usually clear, because a shunt produces a hyperdynamic ventricle, whereas myocardial disease results in hypokinetic function. Looking at how vigorously the ventricle functions will give a strong hint as to the nature of the problem.

A possible reason for hyperdynamic heart failure without a cardiac defect is an arteriovenous malformation, leading to a large arteriovenous shunt. Physiologically, the effect is similar to a combination of an atrial septal defect and a patent ductus arteriosus, because there is a volume load on all cardiac chambers. As a result, we would expect chamber enlargement of all cardiac chambers and hyperdynamic ventricular function. Add this to a normal cardiac survey and the absence of a patent ductus arteriosus, and we have good presumptive evidence to suggest the diagnosis of an arteriovenous malformation.

Hypodynamic cardiac failure can be caused by any disorders that reduce the stroke volume of the heart, including disorders of myocardial function, rhythm disturbances, obstruction to outflow or inflow, and filling disorders. Myocardial disorders as a group are rare in the newborn but may oc-

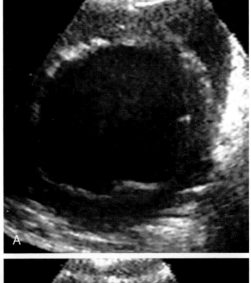

Figure 4–4. These images are from a newborn in the first day of life, with respiratory distress. *A,* A parasternal short-axis view of the left ventricle, which is dilated and hypokinetic. *B,* A high parasternal to suprasternal view showing the ascending aorta and aortic arch. Some vertebral bodies can be seen in the lower right, coursing from the middle right toward the middle bottom of the image. Note the centimeter markers on the right side of the sector. The ascending aorta was only 5 mm in diameter. *C,* A parasternal short-axis view of the tiny aorta in cross-section and the much larger pulmonary artery, which courses downward and bifurcates. This patient had severe aortic stenosis with a hypoplastic ascending aorta and congestive heart failure.

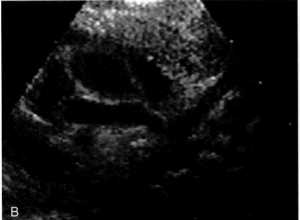

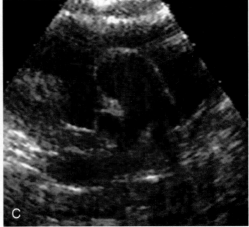

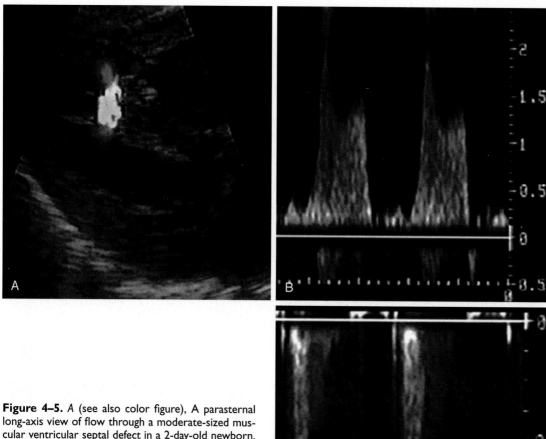

Figure 4–5. *A* (see also color figure), A parasternal long-axis view of flow through a moderate-sized muscular ventricular septal defect in a 2-day-old newborn. *B,* The continuous-wave Doppler recording of the flow shows that there is little pressure difference between the right and left ventricles, because the peak velocity is only 1.9 m/s, or 14 mm Hg. *C,* The tricuspid insufficiency jet, although faint, yields a peak velocity of 3.5 m/s, or 50 mm Hg. We can expect that the symptoms might become more pronounced as the pulmonary vascular resistance falls.

cur. Endocardial fibroelastosis is a disorder of unknown cause that presents an echocardiographic picture of a dilated left ventricle, which is hypocontractile, with increased echogenicity of the endocardium. Myocarditis has numerous causes but appears on echo as left ventricular or biventricular enlargement, without the increased reflectivity of the endocardium. Ischemic disorders are rare, but global ischemia may result

from a difficult resuscitation and appears similar on echocardiography to myocarditis. However, the recovery of function may be more rapid, and the clinical situation should point to the cause. Focal ischemia can occur as a result of either anomalous coronaries or embolic phenomena and is recognized by focal wall motion abnormalities, similar to those seen in adults.

Rhythm disturbances can cause congestive heart failure by reducing effective forward output. If the heart rate is too fast, filling will be impaired, and there can be symptoms of respiratory distress. If the heart rate is too low, there can be an impairment of forward cardiac output, which results in failure as well, although infants and newborns are surprisingly tolerant of moderate bradycardia. In either case, the rhythm disturbance itself should be obvious, and there should be left ventricular dilation as well.

Left-sided failure can be caused by obstruction to outflow (aortic stenosis or coarctation) (Fig. 4–6 [see also color figure] and Fig. 4–4) or rarely by obstruction of inflow (mitral stenosis). The severity of the obstruction can be readily measured by the Doppler estimate of the pressure gradient. In the case of mitral stenosis, the ventricle is normal but the atrium is enlarged. In the case of outflow obstruction as a cause of failure, both will be enlarged, and ventricular contractility will be reduced.

If both the left atrium and left ventricle are normal in size, a cardiac source of failure is unlikely. The remaining cardiac sources of failure can be grouped into restriction of left ventricular filling and restriction of pulmonary venous return. Pericardial effusion can be so significant that it impairs filling of the heart, in which case it

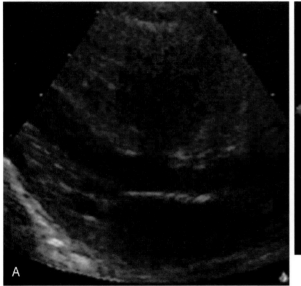

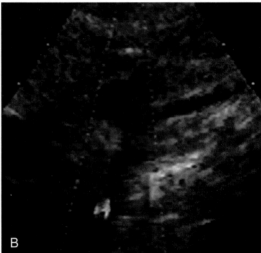

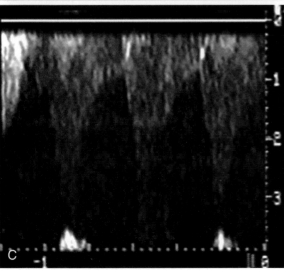

Figure 4–6. These images are from a 10-day-old infant presenting with difficulty feeding. The parasternal long-axis view *(A)* shows a large left atrium and a membranous ventricular septal defect, which was not restrictive. *B* (see also color figure), The color Doppler of the descending aorta, which has a small area of disturbed flow as shown by the green coloration. *C*, The continuous-wave Doppler through that area, with a peak velocity greater than 3 m/s, demonstrating a coarctation as well.

is termed pericardial tamponade. Restrictive myopathy of the left ventricle could lead to failure with normal ventricular size, but the left atrium should be enlarged. Restriction of pulmonary venous return would also lead to poor left ventricular filling and may have high velocities of flow in the left atrium. The most common causes of the rare problem of pulmonary venous restriction are anomalous pulmonary veins, usually of the subcardiac type, and cor triatriatum.

The details of a survey examination sufficient to rule out a cardiac cause of respiratory distress are listed in Box 4–4. Note that the list is much shorter than that in Box 4–3, the potential findings, because most of the findings in Box 4–3 are necessary to fill in the details of the diagnosis. Because we know that most of the cardiac causes of respiratory failure cause left ventricular and left atrial dilation, if neither of these are present, we have narrowed the range of potential causes considerably. The remaining causes are rare but can also be looked for.

Evaluation of an Open Ductus Arteriosus

All newborns have an open ductus arteriosus on the 1st day of life. Because of this, the question in the newly born is seldom whether they have an open ductus arteriosus but rather if the shunt is of physiological significance. At a later age, the mere presence of an open ductus arteriosus is abnormal. As was noted in the section on pulmonary causes of respiratory distress, the respiratory distress itself increases the likelihood that the ductus will remain open or even reopen. In these cases, the evaluation of the contribution of the ductus to the respiratory distress can be difficult. The choice between surgically closing a ductus arteriosus in a critically ill infant or attempting pharmacological closure with indomethacin is made difficult by the high incidence of open ductus in this population and not knowing which infants are likely to actually benefit from the procedure. The echocardiographic examination can provide considerable physiological information to aid this decision. The data can be used to classify the ductal shunt as "physiologically significant," "probably physiologically significant," "not physiologically significant," or "of uncertain physiological significance."

Because there are two types of load for the heart, pressure and volume, we can expect that the consequences of an open ductus can fall into the same categories. The most important for explaining respiratory distress is the volume because it is excessive blood flow through the lungs with elevated venous pressures that causes the fluid build-up and symptoms. If the left atrium and left ventricle are normal in size, it is unlikely that an open ductus arteriosus is the cause of respiratory distress. Similarly, if the velocity of flow through the ductus is high, there must be a low pressure in the pulmonary circulation because there is a significant pressure difference, and the ductus itself must be restrictive to flow. Again, it is unlikely that the ductus is the cause of the respiratory distress. If we see the combination of a ductus, with high flow velocity (>3 m/s) and the chamber dimensions are normal, we should classify the shunt as "not physiologically significant." It is extremely unlikely that closing the ductus arteriosus would significantly improve the condition of the infant (Fig. 4–7 [see also color figure] and Fig. 4–8).

BOX 4–4
SUFFICIENT FINDINGS TO RULE OUT A CARDIAC CAUSE OF RESPIRATORY DISTRESS

Ventricles
  Normal left ventricular size
  Normal left ventricular thickness
  Normal left ventricular function
Atria
  Normal left atrial size
  No extra chamber in left atrium
  No disturbed flow
Other
  No significant pericardial fluid
  Normal rhythm or only sinus tachycardia

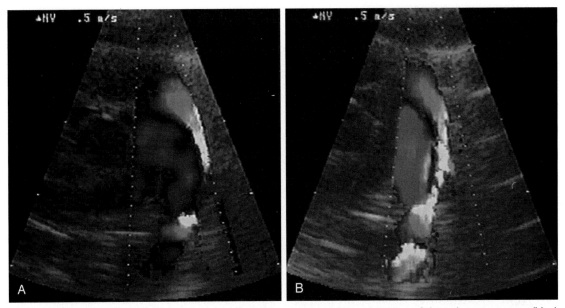

Figure 4–7. *A* (see also color figure), A color Doppler parasternal short-axis view of the pulmonary artery (blue) and its branches as well as the reverse-flow jet through a patent ductus arteriosus. This newborn was 2 days old at the time and had an asymptomatic continuous murmur. Note the location of the jet relative to the pulmonary artery branches. It is overlying the left pulmonary artery, because the ductus is actually to the left and superior to the left pulmonary artery (see Fig. 4–12). *B* (see also color figure), The same ductal flow at a slightly different time in the cardiac cycle, showing how markedly different the color can look for the same physiology.

The opposite is also true. If we find enlargement of the left atrium and left ventricle and there is a low-velocity left-to-right shunt through the ductus, we must classify the ductus as "physiologically significant." There is a high probability that closing the ductus would improve the infant's clinical condition.

If the velocity through the ductus is low, and we see torrential flow from left to right but the ventricle is not enlarged, we should consider the ductus as "probably of physiological significance" whether the left atrium is enlarged or not, because the ventricle may not have had time to dilate (Figs. 4–9 and 4–10). If there is any other combination, the physiology is less clear, and we should consider the flow to be "of uncertain physiological significance" (Table 4–1). In particu-

lar, if the left atrium is not enlarged but there is low velocity flow, we are lacking evidence that the ductus has physiological consequences. This does not mean that it may not be contributing to a difficult clinical situation. It only means that we cannot be certain that closing the ductus will improve the infant's clinical situation. If the pulmonary vascular resistance has not fallen completely, we may obtain this combination of unrestricted flow through a ductus, with a low velocity but no enlargement of chambers. It is common in this situation to have bidirectional shunting, from right to left during systole and left to right during diastole. In this situation as well, the volume load may not be causing problems, although this can change rapidly if the pulmonary vascular resistance falls.

Table 4–1. Classification of Whether a Ductus Arteriosus Is Significant

Variable	Definitely	Probably	Not	Uncertain
Left atrial size	⇑	Normal or ⇑	Normal	All other combinations
Left ventricular size	⇑	Normal	Normal	
Ductal flow velocity	<3 m/s	<3 m/s	>3 m/s	

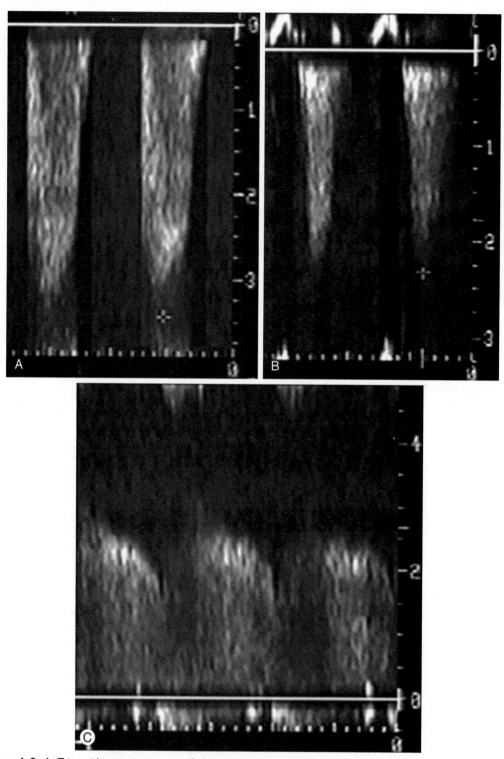

Figure 4–8. *A,* Tricuspid regurgitation in a 2-day-old newborn with a patent ductus arteriosus (PDA) (the same patient as in Figure 4–7). The peak velocity is 3.4 m/s, indicating a right-sided pressure of at least 46 mm Hg, which is elevated. *B,* The tricuspid velocity in the same patient when he was 2 weeks old, with a peak velocity of 2.3 m/s, corresponding to a pressure of 21 mm Hg, which is normal. *C,* The PDA flow in that patient at 2 weeks of age, with a peak velocity of 3.1 m/s, indicating an aortic-to-pulmonary gradient of 38 mm Hg. These findings, along with a small left atrium and left ventricle, indicate that this is a restrictive PDA, which is unlikely to be of physiological significance.

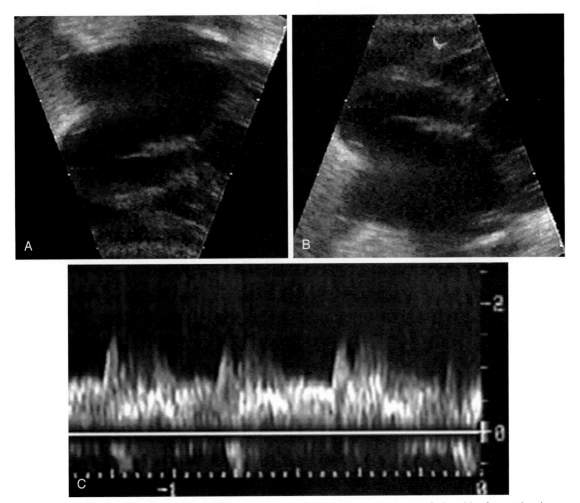

Figure 4–9. *A* and *B*, A subcostal four-chamber view of an enlarged left atrium in a 2-day-old infant with a large, unrestrictive ductus in the standard "pediatric" and "adult" orientations, respectively. The ductal flow velocity is low *(C)*. This ductus is probably of physiological significance.

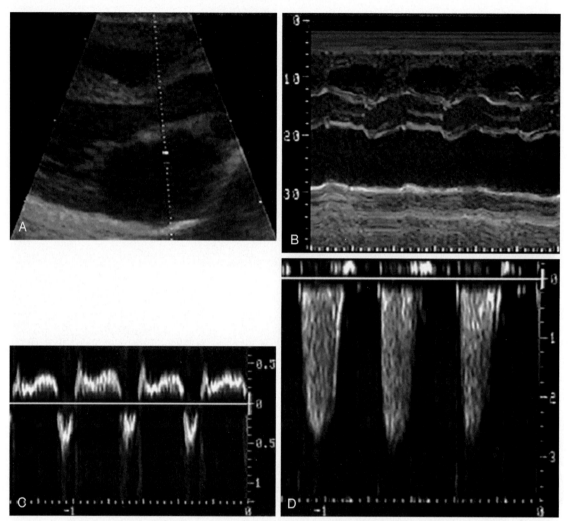

Figure 4–10. A 2-day-old premature newborn with respiratory distress has a large left atrium on two-dimensional imaging *(A)* and M-mode *(B)*, with a left atrium twice the diameter of the aorta. The ductal flow, measured with high-pulse-repetition-frequency Doppler, is bidirectional and of low velocity *(C)*, whereas the tricuspid insufficiency jet is at least 3.0 m/s. *D*, This is an open ductus that is probably hemodynamically significant, but the pulmonary vascular resistance has not fallen completely.

Another finding that indicates hemodynamic significance of a ductus arteriosus is flow reversal in the descending aorta during diastole. In the absence of other causes of flow reversal (aortic insufficiency, aortopulmonary window), this indicates that there is a large flow from left to right through the open ductus (Fig. 4–11; see also color figure).

An anatomic feature worthy of note is the normal position of the ductus arteriosus. It is natural to think that the ductus is located exactly between the right and left pulmonary arteries, but this is not the case. It is normally located superior and to the left of the bifurcation. An easy way to remember

this is the "right-hand rule." If you hold your right hand out with the thumb, index, and middle fingers extended and the palm down, the orientation is similar to the right pulmonary artery, ductus arteriosus, and left pulmonary artery looking from the front of the patient (Fig. 4–12).

When there is right-to-left shunting, the situation is very different. For this to occur, there must be more than just an open ductus because there must be an elevation of the pulmonary pressure to allow this reversal of shunt. Detecting the shunt can be more difficult as well because there will not be an easily visible retrograde flow jet in the pulmonary artery. The key finding is the

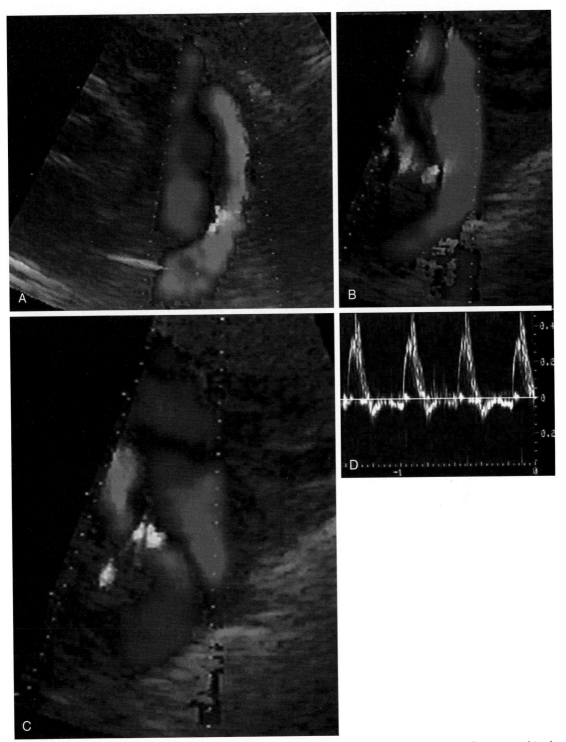

Figure 4–11. Another indication of hemodynamic significance for a patent ductus arteriosus is flow reversal in the descending aorta. A (see also color figure), A parasternal short-axis view of the color flow of a nonrestrictive ductus arteriosus, demonstrated by the lack of evidence for flow acceleration or turbulence. B (see also color figure), A suprasternal view of the aortic arch, with anterograde flow in the descending aorta (blue) and retrograde flow (red) in the ductus arteriosus during systole. C (see also color figure), The same view in diastole, with retrograde flow (red) from the descending aorta distal to the ductus, into the ductus. D, The pulsed Doppler recording from the descending abdominal aorta in the same patient, demonstrating holodiastolic flow reversal (flow away from the transducer).

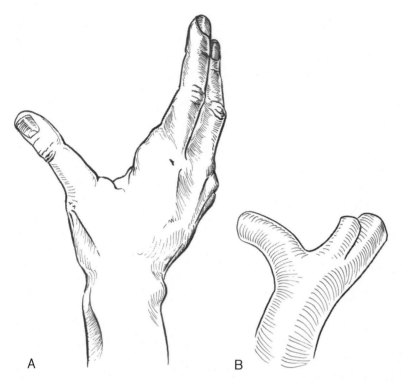

Figure 4–12. The normal position of the ductus is not directly between the right and left pulmonary arteries but rather superior and to the left. This is similar to the position of the index finger when the right hand is held in a relaxed, outstretched position *(A)*. The thumb represents the right pulmonary artery, the middle finger the left pulmonary artery, and the wrist and hand the main pulmonary artery *(B)*.

A

B

elevation of right-sided pressures, as identified by tricuspid regurgitation and pulmonary insufficiency. The degree of elevation and the presence of a right-to-left shunt at the ductal level are the most important findings on the echocardiogram. One should also look for other sources of right-to-left shunting (see Cyanosis). These infants usually have cyanosis as the main presenting problem rather than respiratory distress for reasons outlined under Cyanosis.

The combination of open ductus arteriosus and pulmonary hypertension, with resulting right-to-left shunting and cyanosis, is sometimes called "persistent fetal circulation." Although this term is honored by use, it is rather misleading as to the physiology. "Pulmonary hypertension of the newborn" would perhaps be more descriptive and illuminating. The physiological problem is a high pulmonary vascular resistance, which is nonetheless much lower than during fetal life.

CYANOSIS

Cyanosis is the term used to denote observable desaturation of the circulating blood. The blood that is pumped out the

aorta to the rest of the body is normally fully or almost fully saturated with oxygen because it has just come from the lungs. In a number of conditions, the blood circulating in the body will be less than fully saturated, and this can be observed as a duskiness or even a blueness of the skin. It is most prominent in the mouth (lips, tongue, and gums) and the extremities (fingers and toes). This should be distinguished from circumoral cyanosis, or blueness around the mouth only, and blueness of the fingers and toes, both of which are most often due to vasoconstriction from any cause, such as cold.

Infants can tolerate surprisingly severe desaturation without any apparent distress. This is because they are normally quite desaturated in their fetal life and have special adaptive mechanisms to accomplish efficient oxygen transport, even at these low saturation levels. Perhaps most importantly, they have a special form of hemoglobin, called fetal hemoglobin, with an oxygen dissociation curve that performs well at very low saturations.

Pulmonary Versus Cardiac Disease

There are only two places to look for problems if an infant, or any patient for that matter, is cyanotic: the lungs and the heart. This is because oxygenation occurs in the pulmonary circulation, and the lungs and the heart are only two organs in that circulation.

Cyanosis caused by heart disease means that there is shunting of blood from the unoxygenated systemic venous return to the systemic circulation, or right-to-left shunting. This is not the usual direction of shunting in isolated defects; therefore, the situation must be more complex (see later discussion and Chapter 2 under Cyanosis). Newborns who are cyanotic because of cardiac disease usually do not have any other symptoms because they are able to toleratethe cyanosis well.

Cyanosis from lung disease can occur in one of two ways. The first, intrapulmonary shunting, is similar to cardiac shunting. In this case, there are areas of lung that are not ventilated by air at all but nevertheless have blood flow. Usually the blood flow to an area of lung is reflexly reduced if there is no ventilation, but this mechanism can be imperfect in certain disease states, resulting in blood that passes through the lungs but has not been exposed to air. The second possibility is that the blood has been exposed to air but that the diffusion of oxygen is reduced because of edema, or ventilation is so reduced (hypoventilation) that air is partially trapped and has a low oxygen tension (Box 4–5).

Just as for respiratory distress, there are several differentiating factors between cardiac and noncardiac causes of cyanosis. The infant with a pulmonary cause of cyanosis will be in respiratory distress, probably be-

cause of stimulation of receptors in the lungs. The signs of this respiratory distress include nasal flaring, retractions at the base of the thorax with respiration, and grunting respirations. The presence of these signs suggests that the cause of the cyanosis is pulmonary or has a major pulmonary component.

The other major differentiating factor is that, if diffusion of oxygen or hypoventilation is the problem, allowing the infant to breathe a higher concentration of oxygen will increase the blood oxygen saturation. This will occur within a few minutes in cases of diffusion problems, but only a modest increase will occur if there is a cardiac right-to-left shunt or intrapulmonary shunt. This is because increasing the oxygen concentration in the inspired air will have little effect on the normal pulmonary venous saturation, which is close to 100% anyway, and the shunt will still be there.

It is helpful to determine the most prominent abnormality: respiratory distress or cyanosis. This will suggest whether it is more likely that the cause is pulmonary or cardiac. In spite of this, there is overlap; many types of cardiac defect can cause heart failure, as discussed in the preceding section, which then can cause edema in the lungs, leading to respiratory distress and ultimately cyanosis.

Ruling Out Cardiac Causes of Cyanosis

To have a cardiac cause of cyanosis, there must be right-to-left shunting. As mentioned in Chapter 2, an isolated small or medium-size shunt will result in left-to-right shunting, and this cannot cause cyanosis as the primary presenting sign.

To have right-to-left shunting, there must either be a large defect that would result in equalization of pressures and free bidirectional mixing, or an elevation of right-sided pressures causing a pure right-to-left shunt.

Table 4–2 lists the potential findings that would help explain the cyanosis, subdivided as to whether the predominant mechanism is a large defect with mixing or a smaller

---

BOX 4–5
CAUSES OF CYANOSIS

Pulmonary
  Diffusion defect
  Hypoventilation
  Intrapulmonary shunt
Cardiac
  Right-to-left shunt
  Cardiac failure (diffusion)
Noncardiopulmonary

Table 4–2. Potential Findings in Cardiac Cause of Cyanosis

Variable	Large Defect	Increased Right Pressures
Ventricles	Large discrepancy in size Large ventricular septal defect	Normal size Restrictive defect with right-to-left shunt
Atria	Large atrial septal defect Absent atrial septum	Right atrium larger than left Atrial septum bows to left
Atrioventricular valves	One valve absent Both valves in same ventricle Valves at same level	Severe tricuspid regurgitation Tricuspid displaced to apex (Ebstein's anomaly)
Semilunar valves	Overriding aorta Pulmonic atresia Both from one ventricle	Pulmonic stenosis
Great arteries	Truncus arteriosus Transposition	Peripheral pulmonic stenosis
Right ventricular pressure	Right equals left	Right equal to or greater than left

defect with elevation of the right-sided pressures caused by another defect.

Look for two ventricles, and examine the interventricular septum. Possible causes of cyanosis here would be a large ventricular septal defect, absent interventricular septum, or single ventricle. Septal defects that could be large enough to cause cyanosis include the perimembranous, muscular, and inlet types (Fig. 4–13). The supracristal type of ventricular septal defect rarely causes cyanosis. If there is increased right-sided pressures, a restrictive defect can cause right-to-left shunting, hence the importance of the right ventricular pressure estimate in the survey.

Look for two atria and the interatrial septum. Atrial septal defects that could cause cyanosis include secundum, primum, and sinus venosus defects, but all of these must be very large to cause cyanosis or must be combined with another abnormality that will raise right atrial pressure. This includes tricuspid atresia (Fig. 4–14), Ebstein's anomaly (see Fig. 5–11), and pulmonic atresia, to name a few.

Look at the relative size of the ventricles and atria. If there is anomalous pulmonary venous drainage into the right atrium, either partial or total, this will create a volume load on the right side of the heart, and the right atrium and ventricle will be larger

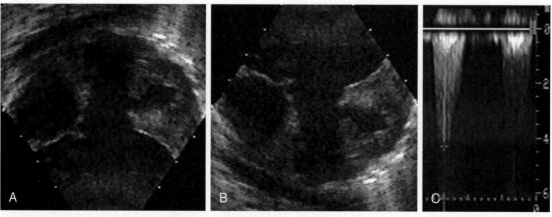

Figure 4–13. These images come from a 2-week-old infant who presented with cyanosis. The first two images are identical subcostal views, presented in the "pediatric" (A) and "adult" (B) orientations. They show a large ventricular septal defect and a large discrepancy in ventricular size. C, The continuous-wave Doppler recording through the pulmonic valve, demonstrating a step-up from the proximal velocity (0.9 m/s) to the peak velocity (4.4 m/s) as marked by the cursors, with a calculated gradient of 74 mm Hg. This patient has both a large ventricular septal defect and pulmonic stenosis with elevation of right ventricular pressure.

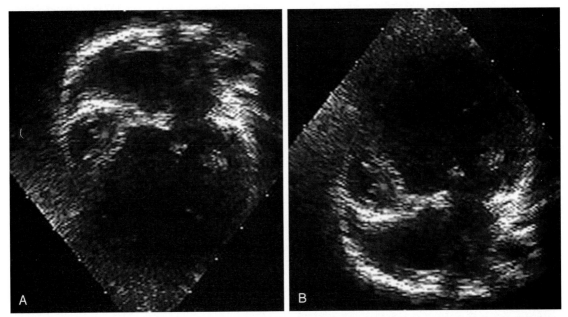

Figure 4–14. This cyanotic newborn has tricuspid atresia, as demonstrated in the standard "pediatric" four-chamber view *(A)* and the "adult" four-chamber view *(B)*. Note the absence of a tricuspid valve and the small right ventricular chamber, which communicates with the large left ventricle through a large ventricular septal defect, which is out of the plane of the image.

than normal. Partial anomalous pulmonary veins can cause an elevation of the right atrial pressures and a resulting pressure gradient that may drive a right-to-left shunt through a patent foramen ovale, causing cyanosis. In total anomalous pulmonary veins, there must be a right-to-left shunt at some level for the infant to have survived, and there is complete mixing of the pulmonary

and systemic venous return, causing cyanosis.

Look at the relationship of the two atrioventricular valves, in particular whether one is absent (atretic, as in Fig. 4–14), whether each drains into a different ventricle, and whether they happen to be at the same level as in an atrioventricular septal defect (Fig. 4–15). An atrioventricular sep-

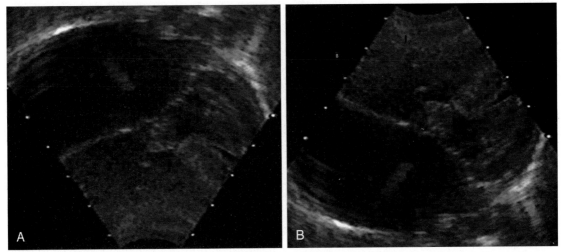

Figure 4–15. These almost apical four-chamber images are from a 7-month-old with cyanosis. The images are identical, differing only in the orientation. *A,* "Pediatric" orientation. *B,* The "adult" orientation. Note the primum atrial septal defect, the straddling atrioventricular valves, both of which are on the same level, and the inlet ventricular septal defect, with partial occlusion by redundant valvular tissue.

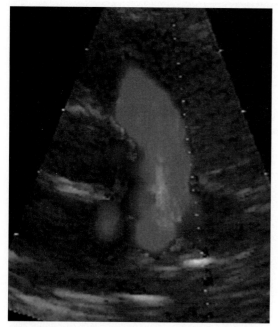

Figure 4–16 (see also color figure). Parasternal view of the normal crossing of the pulmonary artery and the aorta in a 2-month-old. The pulmonary artery flow is visible as blue, flowing away from the transducer toward the lungs. The aorta is visible running from the midportion on the left down and to the right, passing behind the pulmonary artery. Note how the two arteries cross almost perpendicularly.

tal defect often results in bidirectional shunting of blood at either the atrial or the ventricular level. The relative position of the valves can also be exaggerated. In Ebstein's anomaly the tricuspid valve is markedly displaced toward the apex of the ventricle, and there is significant tricuspid insufficiency and resulting right-to-left shunting through the foramen ovale and cyanosis.

Look for the great arteries and semilunar valves, and make sure they are connected to the correct ventricle (Fig. 4–16 [see also color figure] and Fig. 4–17). In transposition of the great arteries, the infant may be clinically cyanotic in some cases and will definitely have unsaturated circulating blood. Also, many of the more complex lesions may include transposition. There may be only one great artery (truncus arteriosus) (Fig. 4–18), or both of the arteries may come from the same ventricle, known as double-outlet right or left ventricle. There may be severe hypoplasia or stenosis of one of the great vessels and associated semilunar valve. One particularly common combination is pulmonic stenosis with malalignment ventricular septal defect and the aortic valve overriding the defect. This is called tetralogy of Fallot and is discussed later under Syndromes.

Look for an open ductus arteriosus. We may see a large ductus at this point, although right-to-left shunting causing cyanosis is often difficult to visualize. A left-to-right shunt could cause respiratory distress and rarely secondary cyanosis.

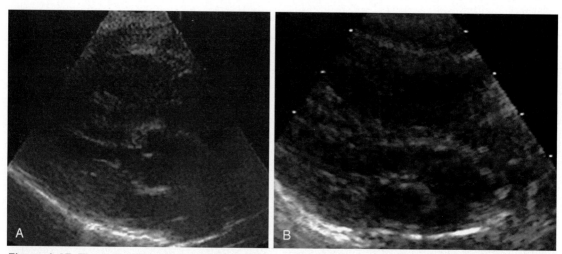

Figure 4–17. These two parasternal long-axis images are from different 1-day-olds with transposition of the great arteries. A, The aortic and pulmonary valves are visible in the same plane in the same orientation. This is not possible in normals. It is also possible to see the pulmonary artery, which is originating from the left ventricle on the bottom of the image, coursing posteriorly shortly after its origin. B, A similar view, showing the beginning of the pulmonary bifurcation.

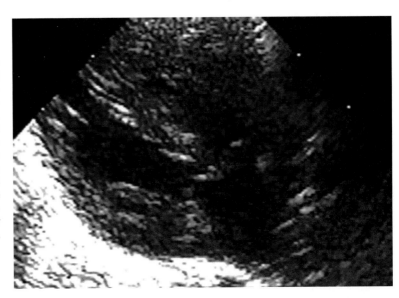

Figure 4–18. This cyanotic newborn has a large great vessel that is overriding the ventricular septum; hence, this is a malalignment ventricular septal defect. This is a parasternal long-axis view: the cusps of the great vessel meet exactly over the ventricular septum, meaning that this would be classified as a 50% override. This view is compatible with a number of defects, including (but not limited to) tetralogy of Fallot and truncus arteriosus, which is what this patient had.

If a large defect is not found in the survey outlined previously, there may be an elevation of right-sided pressures leading to right-to-left shunting through a smaller defect. Right-sided pressures can be estimated in several ways.

The foremost of these is to estimate the right ventricular systolic pressure by measuring the velocity of tricuspid regurgitation. Using the simplified Bernoulli equation, we can then calculate the estimated right ventricular to right atrial pressure difference. Right atrial pressure is a variable in the final estimate of right ventricular pressure, but the range of variation of right atrial pressure is much less than that of right ventricular pressure. Thus, we can estimate the right ventricular systolic pressure to within 10 to 15 mm Hg in most cases without estimating the right atrial pressure.

Another way of estimating the right ventricular and pulmonary artery pressures is to measure the pulmonary insufficiency velocity. The right ventricular diastolic pressure is similar to the right atrial pressures, and the same arguments apply to the pulmonary artery to right ventricular diastolic gradient as to the right ventricular to right atrial systolic gradient. The early diastolic pulmonary artery pressure is similar to the mean pulmonary artery pressure and, if elevated, indicates that the right ventricular systolic pressure must be elevated as well.

If the right ventricular pressure is not

elevated, we know that there cannot be right-to-left shunting at the ventricular or arterial level. This is because we cannot have a pressure gradient that would drive the flow, nor can there be such a large defect that there would be equalization of pressures and bidirectional mixing. Similarly, if the pulmonary artery pressure is not elevated, we cannot have right-to-left ductal flow.

At the atrial level, assessment of the pressure relationships is not as straightforward. If we can see some bowing of the interatrial septum, the direction of bowing will tell us about the pressure relationships. Bowing to the right is normal because the pressure in the left atrium is generally higher than in the right. Bowing to the left indicates an elevation of the right atrial pressure relative to the left atrial pressure and the possibility of a right-to-left shunt through a restrictive defect.

Box 4–6 lists the details of the survey examination sufficient to rule out a cardiac cause of cyanosis. If all of the anatomic structures are grossly intact and there is no evidence for elevation of the right-sided pressures, we have ruled out a cardiac cause of cyanosis.

SHOCK

Shock is defined as a condition in which there is inadequate perfusion of the body. It

> **BOX 4–6**
> **SUFFICIENT FINDINGS TO RULE**
> **OUT A CARDIAC CAUSE OF**
> **CYANOSIS**
>
> Ventricles
>   Equal in size
>   No large ventricular septal defect
> Atria
>   Equal in size
>   Interatrial septum without large defects
>   Interatrial septum does not bow to left
> Atrioventricular valves
>   Each empties into respective ventricle
>   No significant tricuspid regurgitation
>   Tricuspid only slightly displaced toward
>   apex of ventricle
> Semilunar valves/great arteries
>   Both present, similar in size, and from
>   respective ventricles
> Right ventricular pressure estimate
>   Right ventricle less than left ventricle

Shock is always a medical emergency because the inadequate perfusion, if not corrected promptly, can lead to serious and potentially permanent damage to organs such as the brain, kidneys, liver, and gut. From the prior description, it should be clear that there is a close relationship between the physiology of shock and congestive heart failure. Both can have a "hypodynamic" type and a "hyperdynamic" type. There are many clinical diagnoses in which shock or congestive heart failure, or both, can result. Also, the clinical presentation can be very similar. Both can present with a prominent finding of respiratory distress.

Different Profiles of Noncardiac Shock

If there is nothing intrinsically wrong with the heart or valves, it is still possible to have a low cardiac output causing shock. This occurs if there is inadequate filling of the heart chambers. This is most commonly due to either hypovolemia (low circulating blood volume) or an obstruction to venous return. In either case, the cardiac chambers, which are underfilled, are small, and cardiac contraction is vigorous.

If the filling of the heart is normal, then hypovolemia cannot be present, and the only other cause of noncardiac shock is severe peripheral vasodilation, which causes a low blood pressure in the presence of a high cardiac output. The most common cause for a lowered peripheral vascular resistance causing noncardiac shock is certain forms of sepsis, especially gram-negative sepsis. This is such a common relation that shock from peripheral vasodilation is often called "septic shock." However, the shock caused by sepsis, even gram-negative sepsis, can be due to hypovolemia or decreased cardiac function as well.

can occur in one of two ways: (1) when there is inadequate cardiac output, sometimes called low output shock, and (2) when there is an adequate output but peripheral vasodilation so severe that the blood flow is poorly distributed and some vital organs are not receiving an adequate blood supply. This latter is sometimes called high-output shock. In either case, the blood pressure will be quite low. Inadequate cardiac output can be further subdivided into cardiac causes and inadequate filling of a normal heart (hypovolemia). Each of the resulting three physiological subdivisions has a different profile on echocardiographic examination (Table 4–3).

Table 4–3. Findings in Different Physiological Types of Shock

Variable	Hypovolemic	Vasodilatory	Cardiac
LA and LV size	Small	Normal or small	Large or structural defect (see Box 4–7)
LV function	⇑	Normal or ⇑	⇓

LA, left atrium; LV, left ventricle.

In the case of shock from peripheral vaso-dilation, we would also expect that there may be dilation of all four cardiac chambers and hyperdynamic ventricular function. The patient will almost always be showing other signs of illness, which may include hypoto-nia and respiratory distress.

Although it seems obvious, it bears men-tioning that in these cases the treatment of the shock itself is merely supportive, not curative, and the patient needs treatment for the primary cause of the low peripheral vascular resistance.

The hallmarks of a noncardiac cause of shock are hyperdynamic cardiac function with small to mildly enlarged chambers.

Cardiac Diagnosis When the Cause Is Cardiac

For a heart problem to cause shock, it must result in a low cardiac output. We have already examined the noncardiac rea-sons for a low output—obstruction to venous return or hypovolemia—and, fortunately, the cardiac causes are relatively limited as well. The potential findings are listed in Box 4–7. Note the similarity to the potential findings in respiratory failure, listed in Box 4–3. Other conditions that do not cause heart failure can cause shock, however. These are extreme expressions of cyanosis, in which there is severely inadequate oxy-genation, even though perfusion is inade-quate. Shock in these cases results from reflex vasodilation. This can be due to any of the causes of cyanosis, including transpo-sition of the great arteries and the more severe forms of tetralogy and pulmonary atresia.

A diminished cardiac output sufficient to cause shock can be caused by decreased myocardial function or obstruction to flow. Myocardial function can be divided into sys-tolic function and diastolic function. In the infant, it is most often systolic function that is diminished as a result of heart block, supraventricular tachycardia, myocardial ischemia, or other injury such as toxins or myocarditis. Diastolic function can be di-minished as a result of hypertrophy (second-ary to another condition or primary) or ex-

BOX 4–7
POTENTIAL FINDINGS ON EXAMINATION FOR CARDIAC CAUSE OF SHOCK

Ventricles
  Dilated left ventricle
  Hypoplastic left ventricle
Atria
  Dilated left atrium
  Atrioventricular valves
  Mitral stenosis
Semilunar valves
  Aortic stenosis
Great arteries
  Coarctation of the aorta
  Transposition
Right ventricular pressure estimate
  Normal or slight increase
Other
  Pericardial effusion
  Severe bradycardia
  Severe tachycardia

ternal problems such as pericardial effusion with tamponade. An additional possibility is that the infant has no functional left ven-tricle and that when the ductus begins to close there is a loss of effective circulation. This occurs in the hypoplastic left heart syn-drome. In transposition of the great arter-ies, there is also this ductal dependency, except there may be effective circulation, but the blood is not adequately oxygenated. This can either present as cyanosis or shock, depending on the degree of reflex vasodila-tion.

Obstructions to flow consist of all of the "pressure load" conditions listed under Car-diac Causes of Respiratory Distress. These include all types of valvular stenosis and peripheral obstructions such as coarctation.

These possible causes lead directly to a sequence of looking for these problems. If systolic function is diminished, we should see chamber dilation and decreased motion or a greatly reduced or increased heart rate.

> **BOX 4–8**
> **SUFFICIENT FINDINGS TO RULE**
> **OUT A CARDIAC CAUSE OF SHOCK**
>
> Ventricles
>   Both of normal size
> Atria
>   Left atrium normal size
> Great arteries/semilunar valves
>   Equal size
>   No transposition
> Other
>   No significant pericardial fluid
>   Normal rhythm or only sinus tachycardia

Either of these should be clear on the initial examination of the heart. Similarly, if there are any ductal dependent forms of shock, we should see either gross hypoplasia of the left ventricle or transposition of the great arteries. Diastolic dysfunction should be considered if there is a pericardial effusion or myocardial hypertrophy.

In summary, we should look for differential enlargement of cardiac chambers, decreased systolic function, very high or low heart rate, or external compression of the heart. If none of these are present, a cardiac cause of shock cannot be supported (Box 4–8).

ASYMPTOMATIC INFANT WITH A MURMUR

A fairly frequent finding is that an otherwise healthy infant has a murmur noted on examination in the hospital. This is a very different situation from the infant who is cyanotic, is in shock, or has congestive heart failure or respiratory distress. As a result, the spectrum of possible disorders is quite different, and the examination can be directed at the potential findings for this situation. The potential findings on the examination for an asymptomatic murmur are listed in Box 4–9.

Functional Sources of Murmur in the Newborn

Newborns have many sources for transient murmurs that have no clinical consequences or long-term effects. All of the most common can be understood in terms of the changes that occur after birth and in the first few months of life. The most common of the nonpathological murmur types are ductus arteriosus murmurs, tricuspid insufficiency murmurs, and pulmonary flow murmur of the newborn.

All newborns have an open ductus arteriosus. This tends to narrow immediately, but complete closure may take 48 hours or longer. The usual murmur from a ductus arteriosus is continuous and often described as sounding like running machinery. In the newborn, however, the murmur of a ductus may sometimes be heard predominantly in systole. The findings of a ductus arteriosus on echocardiographic examination have been discussed in the evaluation of the duc-

> **BOX 4–9**
> **POTENTIAL FINDINGS ON**
> **EXAMINATION FOR ASYMPTOMATIC**
> **MURMUR**
>
> Ventricles
>   Small ventricular septal defect
> Atria
>   Atrial septal defect
> Atrioventricular valves
>   Tricuspid regurgitation
>   Mitral regurgitation
> Semilunar valves
>   Pulmonic stenosis
>   Aortic stenosis
> Great vessels
>   Ductus arteriosus
>   Coarctation
>   Disturbed flow in branch pulmonary
>   arteries
> Right ventricular pressure
>   Elevated (may cause false-negative
>   examination)

tus arteriosus. Two points are worth repeating here. First, the velocity of flow through the ductus is a function of the pressure difference, and the pulmonary pressure in a newborn is elevated soon after birth, dropping rapidly during the following hours and days. This means that the examination can also change rapidly, leading to more or less dramatic findings. A ductus that may be difficult to find in the 1st day of life because of small pressure differences between the pulmonary and systemic circulations may become very easy to identify 1 day later when the pressure differences are larger and resulting velocities are higher. That it is easy to identify does not mean that it has become worse. In fact, this may be a sign that it is less important because it is restricting flow and creating a pressure drop.

Second, because there are such major changes in the first few days, the threshold for intervention in an infant who is doing well should be high. Some believe that intervention for an open ductus arteriosus, for example, in this situation is never warranted. The echocardiographic examination, therefore, is directed at identifying the source of the murmur, characterizing the physiology, and looking for other pathology.

The next kind of functional murmur of the newborn is quite common and is also related to the changes in right-sided pressures that occur soon after birth. The tricuspid valve is often insufficient in normal infants, children, and adults. Estimates of the incidence of tricuspid insufficiency in normal individuals range as high as 80%. Soon after birth, the pressure in the right ventricle is still high, so that the velocity of this insufficiency is high. Because the tricuspid valve is the closest to the chest wall, this may be audible at the lower sternal border on the right or left as a systolic murmur. On echocardiographic examination, everything is normal, including a "normal" tricuspid insufficiency, with a high velocity because of the elevated right-sided pressures. If the infant is re-examined in 24 hours, the pressures will usually have gone down, with a resulting reduction in velocities, and the murmur will be reduced in intensity or will have disappeared.

The last major cause of a functional murmur in the newborn is the pulmonary flow murmur of the newborn. The ratio of the branch pulmonary artery size to main pulmonary artery size in the newborn infant is smaller than at any other age. This is because the main pulmonary artery had a considerable flow in the fetal period, mostly traveling through the ductus to the body, whereas the flow through the branch pulmonary arteries was very limited. In some infants, this disproportion is sufficient to cause some turbulence of blood flow through the branch pulmonary arteries, although there is no significant gradient. The murmur is heard best over the lung fields, much like peripheral pulmonary stenosis, from which it is indistinguishable on clinical examination.

The echocardiographic examination is diagnostic, showing a slight acceleration of flow through the branch pulmonary arteries as well as no significant elevation of the right-sided pressures as estimated by tricuspid regurgitation or pulmonary regurgitation (Fig. 4–19; see also color figure). In the case of a real peripheral pulmonic stenosis, there would be a significant elevation of the right-sided pressures, although the site of the narrowing may or may not be visible on the echocardiographic examination. It should be noted that even if a site of narrowing is visualized, there may be others outside of the range of the echocardiographic windows.

Typically, a follow-up examination of such an infant at 6 months of age shows completely normal flow in the pulmonary arteries, and the murmur is no longer heard.

Cardiac Defects

In this case, we are looking for the cardiac causes of an asymptomatic murmur, which limits the range of severity considerably. I have already mentioned some of the cardiac causes of murmur in the previous section, because they are transitory and not to be considered defects. Here I consider true cardiac defects.

Asymptomatic cardiac murmurs are usually caused by a ventricular septal defect

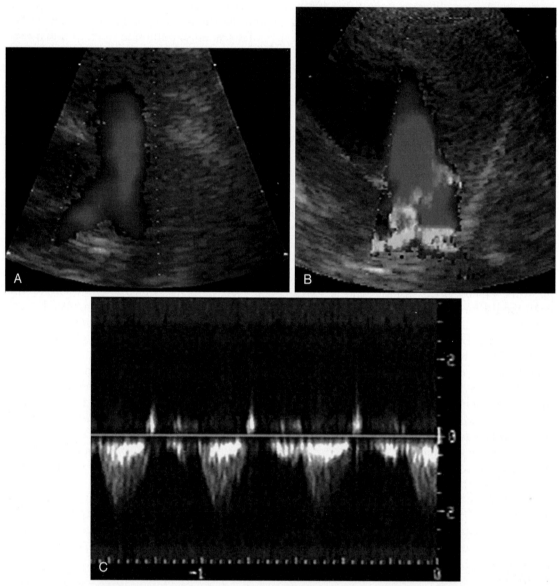

Figure 4–19. *A* (see also color figure), Color flow Doppler of the main pulmonary artery and branches of a normal 1-week-old infant. Note that there is no disturbed flow. *B* (see also color figure), The color flow Doppler of the main pulmonary artery and branches of a 1-month-old infant with a systolic murmur radiating to the lungs. There is disturbed flow at both of the branch points. Using high-pulse-repetition-frequency Doppler, it is possible to quantitate the degree of obstruction, as is done in *C*. This measurement from the left pulmonary artery shows a peak velocity of 2.0 m/s, which indicates that even if we were to consider this a stenosis, the peak gradient would be less than 16 mm Hg. In fact, this is the result of a normal variant, with relative narrowing of the origin of the right and left pulmonary arteries, and this is a functional pulmonary flow murmur.

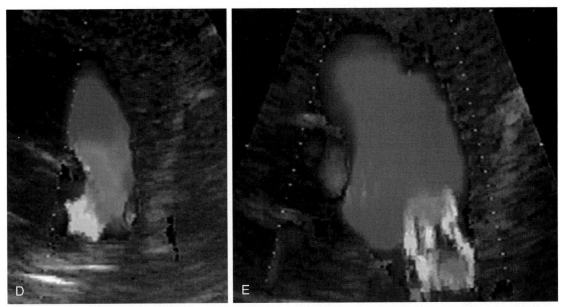

Figure 4–19 *Continued.* It does not always affect both sides. It can affect only the right *(D;* see also color figure) or the left side *(E;* see also color figure).

(Figs. 4–20 and 4–21; see also color figures), pulmonic stenosis (Fig. 4–22), aortic stenosis (Fig. 4–23), ductus arteriosus, or rarely atrial septal defect (Fig. 4–24). Each of these should be readily detectable on the transthoracic examination.

In any case, one must be careful when assessing the severity of any of these lesions. Because of the large physiological changes that occur in the perinatal period, the physiology observed on one day may radically change within a few days. The most important changes are shifts in the pulmonary vascular resistance. These are high shortly after birth, leading to elevated pulmonary pressures.

This means that a ductus arteriosus or ventricular septal defect may appear to be of little significance early on, because the pulmonary resistance and pressure are high, leading to very little shunting. When the pressures are equal, the flow may be absent at first, making detection almost impossible unless we can identify the duct on two-dimensional examination. Later, when the pulmonary vascular resistance falls, the shunt would increase in magnitude, making detection easier. The way to avoid mistakenly "ruling out" a ductus when it is actually present is to estimate the pulmonary artery pressure, using either the tricuspid

insufficiency jet velocity or the pulmonic insufficiency velocity. If the right-sided pressures are high, a significant duct may be missed.

Peripheral pulmonic stenosis can be difficult to diagnose on echocardiographic examination because the narrowed portions of the pulmonary arteries may not be visible. The key is the typical systolic murmur, which is best heard over the lung fields, and the elevation of right-sided pressures on echocardiographic examination.

Caveats (What You Could Miss)

The main caveat when evaluating a murmur in the newborn is that the severity of the discovered lesion can vary dramatically with the physiological changes after birth, although there are others as well that are discussed at the end of this section. As noted, the pulmonary vascular resistance drops soon after birth, resulting in lower pulmonary vascular pressures and higher flows through the pulmonary circulation. A few examples of how this can alter the assessment of severity of a lesion will serve to illustrate the problem.

Pulmonic stenosis found in a newborn in the first few days of life may increase in

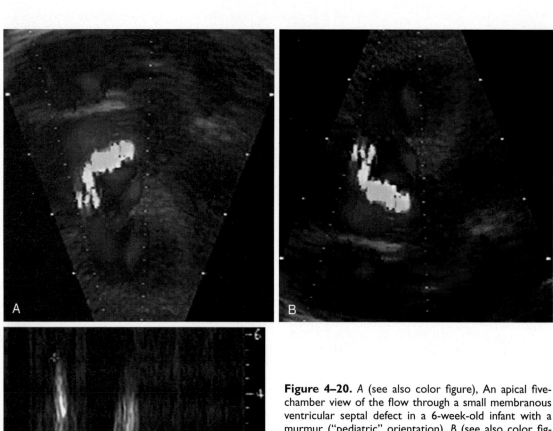

Figure 4–20. *A* (see also color figure), An apical five-chamber view of the flow through a small membranous ventricular septal defect in a 6-week-old infant with a murmur ("pediatric" orientation). *B* (see also color figure), The same image in the "adult" orientation. The continuous-wave Doppler recording *(C)* shows that the peak velocity is 5.2 m/s, yielding a pressure gradient of 108 mm Hg, showing that this is a restrictive ventricular septal defect.

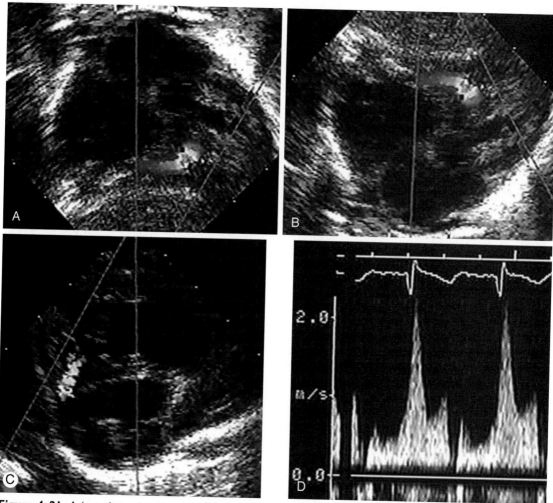

Figure 4–21. *A* (see also color figure), A posteriorly angled subcostal four-chamber view taken from a newborn with a systolic murmur (standard "pediatric" orientation). *B* (see also color figure), The same image in the "adult" orientation. There is evidence of disturbed flow across the ventricular septum, from the left to the right ventricle. *C* (see also color figure), The short-axis view on the same patient demonstrating the posterior location of the small muscular ventricular septal defect. *D*, The Doppler recording of the flow through the defect, which shows the peculiar pattern of the flow being reduced in midsystole as a result of the contraction of the surrounding muscle. This is a sign that the channel is quite small.

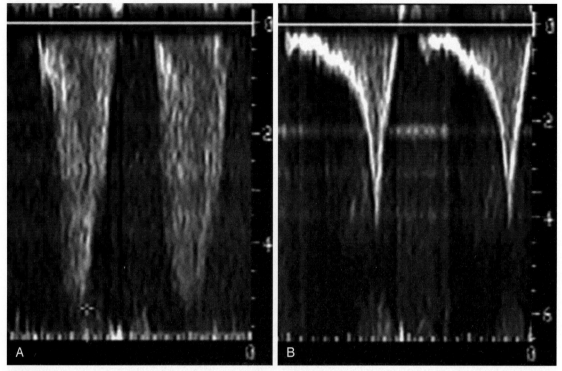

Figure 4–22. *A*, The continuous-wave Doppler of the pulmonic valve flow in a 4-month-old infant with a murmur and valvular pulmonic stenosis. The peak velocity is 5.2 m/s, yielding a pressure gradient of 108 mm Hg. *B*, The high-pulse-repetition-frequency Doppler just below the pulmonic valve, demonstrating a muscular obstruction in the right ventricular outflow tract and a late-peaking, high-velocity flow. The late-peak velocity is 4.2 m/s, or 70 mm Hg.

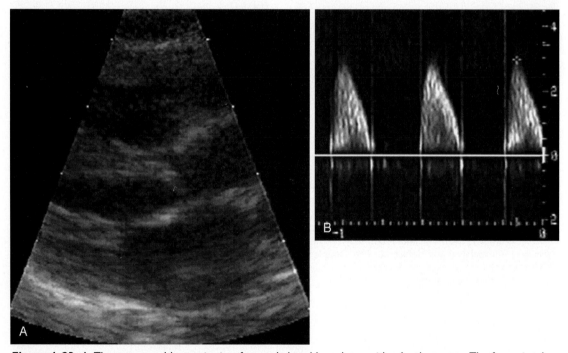

Figure 4–23. *A*, The parasternal long-axis view from a 1-day-old newborn with a loud murmur. The frame is taken in systole, and there is doming of the aortic valve as well as mild poststenotic dilatation of the ascending aorta. The left atrium is also dilated, being almost twice the size of the aortic root. *B*, The continuous-wave Doppler recording through the aortic valve in the same patient. The peak velocity (marked by the cursor) is 3.0 m/s, yielding a peak calculated gradient of 36 mm Hg.

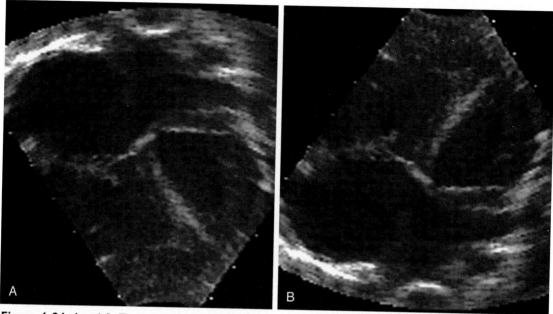

Figure 4–24. *A* and *B*, These images are identical but are shown in different orientations. Both are apical four-chamber views from a 6-month-old with a murmur. *A*, "Pediatric" orientation. *B*, "Adult" orientation. Note that the atrioventricular valves are at the same level and that there is a primum atrial septal defect but no ventricular septal defect.

apparent severity as the pulmonary vascular resistance falls and pulmonary forward flow increases. This is due not to an increased narrowing of the valve but rather to an increase in forward flow. Similarly, but by another mechanism, the severity of a coarctation can change dramatically as the ductus closes. In this case, it is probably a real change in the severity of the narrowing rather that just a change in the flows.

If we detect a ventricular septal defect, the apparent severity can change as well because the pressure in the right ventricle will be high soon after birth and decrease later. We may find little calculated shunt, with a low Qp:Qs, but the ventricular septal defect may still be large. Clearly, if the defect is easily visible, we can more readily assess the true size and physiological significance even before the pulmonary vascular resistance has fallen.

Because of this, there is no way to assess reliably the severity of many lesions before the pulmonary vascular resistance has fallen and the ductus is closed. This also points the way to our solution: that we should not make a final assessment of severity until the pulmonary vascular resis-

tance has fallen (if it is going to!) and the ductus arteriosus has closed.

One point that sometimes causes confusion is the relationship between severity of a lesion and the velocity of flow across it. A common misunderstanding is that low-velocity flow across a ventricular septal defect or patent ductus arteriosus means that the lesion is of little significance, whereas high-velocity flow is more significant. Exactly the opposite is true. With a high-velocity flow, the lesion is restrictive to flow and there is a significant pressure difference. With a low-velocity flow, either the flow is unrestricted, in which case the lesion is highly significant, or the pulmonary vascular resistance has not yet fallen and the significance is difficult to assess.

There are also some lesions that are difficult to detect in the newborn period but are also of limited clinical significance then. The primary example of this is the atrial septal defect (Fig. 4–25; see also color figure). An atrial septal defect may consist of a so-called fenestrated atrial septum, with a net-like membrane over the hole. In this case, the image may not reveal the defect, and the degree of shunting in the newborn

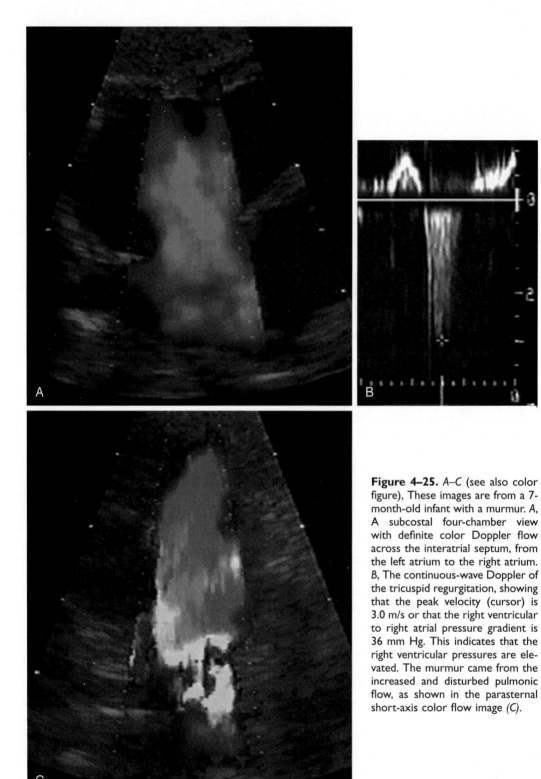

Figure 4–25. A–C (see also color figure), These images are from a 7-month-old infant with a murmur. A, A subcostal four-chamber view with definite color Doppler flow across the interatrial septum, from the left atrium to the right atrium. B, The continuous-wave Doppler of the tricuspid regurgitation, showing that the peak velocity (cursor) is 3.0 m/s or that the right ventricular to right atrial pressure gradient is 36 mm Hg. This indicates that the right ventricular pressures are elevated. The murmur came from the increased and disturbed pulmonic flow, as shown in the parasternal short-axis color flow image (C).

BOX 4–10

SUFFICIENT FINDINGS TO RULE OUT A PATHOLOGICAL CARDIAC CAUSE OF ASYMPTOMATIC MURMUR

Ventricles

  No ventricular septal defect flow

Atria

  No atrial septal defect flow

Atrioventricular valves

  No more than moderate tricuspid
    regurgitation

  No more than mild mitral regurgitation

Semilunar valves

  No high-velocity flow in aortic valve

  No high-velocity flow in pulmonic valve

Great vessels

  No patent ductus flow

  No coarctation flow

Right-sided pressure

  Normal

---

period may not be sufficient to be easily detected.

If there are no significant valvular abnormalities, there are no small shunts, and there is no narrowing of either the peripheral pulmonary arteries or the aorta (coarctation), we have ruled out pathological cardiac causes of an asymptomatic murmur (Box 4–10).

SYNDROMES

As mentioned in Chapter 2, syndromes are recognized constellations of defects. There are several clinical reasons for identifying syndromes. The most important is that a given syndrome is associated with a certain prognosis and complications, so identification is important for these reasons as well as communication. The other important reason is that if one has identified a syndrome, there are certain associated anomalies that are highly probable, which can be identified specifically.

What to Look for in Tetralogy of Fallot

Tetralogy of Fallot is perhaps the classic collection of cardiac defects into a syndrome. It consists of pulmonic stenosis, overriding aorta, ventricular septal defect, and right ventricular hypertrophy (Fig. 4–26). Some of the features may not be as prominent in the newborn as later in life. In particular, right ventricular hypertrophy may be indistinguishable from the normal hypertrophy of the newborn right ventricle, and the pulmonic stenosis may not cause as great a gradient as later, for reasons to be explained.

Newborns with tetralogy usually undergo consultation for either cyanosis (hypoxia) or murmur, or both. Often there is a chest x-ray film with the characteristic "boot-shape" ventricle actually caused by the absence of the normal pulmonary artery contour accentuating the apex of the ventricle.

The ventricular septal defect is usually very easy to find. It is in a similar location to a perimembranous ventricular septal defect, and because it is associated with malalignment of the great arteries, it is never a tiny, pinhole defect. There is usually easily detectable flow across the defect during both systole and diastole.

The degree of aortic override is variable. Up to 25% is considered normal. If there is 100% override, the diagnosis changes to double-outlet right ventricle with pulmonic stenosis, assuming that there is pulmonic stenosis and the pulmonary artery is still connected to the right ventricle. The degree of override is also one of the details that determines the degree of cyanosis the patient will have.

The pulmonic stenosis may be purely valvular, which is less common, or may involve some degree of hypoplasia of the main pulmonary artery. This can have very important consequences for the outcome of surgical repair of the defect, because hypoplasia of the main pulmonary artery is more difficult to repair. The severity of the pulmonic stenosis is often difficult to assess in the newborn period because of the physiological changes that are occurring. In particular, pulmonary artery pressure can be

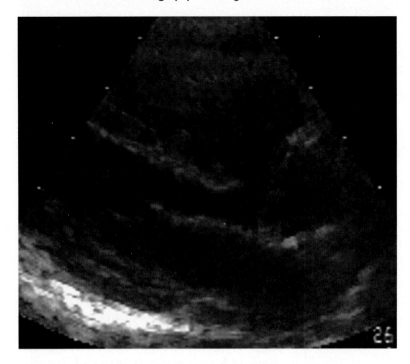

Figure 4–26. This parasternal long-axis view is of a 9-month-old with tetralogy of Fallot. Illustrated here is the malalignment ventricular septal defect, with the aorta overriding at least 50%.

raised, reducing the gradient across the valve.

Two mechanisms can contribute to this elevation of pulmonary artery pressure: (1) the elevation of pulmonary vascular resistance just after birth, and (2) the still-open ductus arteriosus, increasing blood flow through the lungs. We can guard against the error of underestimating the degree of pulmonic stenosis by noting whether the ductus is open or closed and, if it is open, what the velocity of its flow is, and therefore inducing what the pulmonary pressures are. If there is an open ductus with low-velocity flow, we cannot accurately assess the final gradient across the pulmonic valve because the pressures in the pulmonary artery are elevated. If the ductus is narrow and there is a high velocity, we have a better estimate because we know that the pulmonary pressures are low. If the ductus is closed, we must be uncertain because the pulmonary vascular resistance can still be high.

What to Look for in Hypoplastic Left Heart Syndrome

Hypoplastic left heart syndrome usually presents within the 1st week of life, with heart failure or shock. The sudden onset of symptoms is due to the closure of the ductus arteriosus, which results in inadequate blood flow to the systemic circulation.

The echocardiographic diagnosis is usually quite apparent. The left-sided heart structures are all extremely underdeveloped, including the ascending aorta, aortic valve, left ventricle, and mitral valve (see Fig. 3–10). The usual diagnostic criterion is that the ascending aorta is less than 6 mm in diameter, although it is often much smaller. This is the invariant portion of the syndrome; the development of the left ventricle and mitral valve varies. In some cases, the left ventricle may even be dilated (see Fig. 4–4). Other combinations include atresia of the aortic valve with severely hypoplastic ascending aorta and either ventricular septal defect or atrioventricular septal defect.

What to Look for in Atrioventricular Septal Defect

An atrioventricular septal defect usually presents either as cyanosis in a newborn or as part of an evaluation for some other systemic syndrome. The diagnosis is most apparent on the four-chamber views, in which the primum atrial septal defect, inlet ventricular septal defect, and abnormalities of placement and function of the atrioventricular valves are all apparent (see Fig. 4–15).

A subtle but hallmark finding is that the tricuspid and mitral valves are at the same level in the heart. Normally, the tricuspid valve is displaced apically relative to the mitral valve, but in all of the variants in the atrioventricular septal defect complex both valves are at the same level. A word of caution is in order, however. Even in normal individuals, it is possible to create images that give the appearance of both of the atrioventricular valves being at the same level. In a true atrioventricular defect, this appearance will be apparent from all views. The anterior mitral valve leaflet always has a cleft, but this can be difficult to demonstrate in the newborn.

An important issue for the repair of such defect is the extent to which the atrioventricular valves are easily segregated into the respective ventricles. The easiest situation is when each valve and all of its chordal attachments are fully contained within the ventricle in which it belongs. In other patients, however, there may be chords attached to the ridge of the ventricular septal defect or even crossing over into the other ventricle. Both situations are of increasing complexity and difficult to repair.

What to Look for in Coarctation of the Aorta

Coarctation of the aorta often presents as heart failure or shock but may present as a murmur as well. In the initial examination, there can be findings of left ventricular failure, with dilation of the left ventricle or left atrium (see Fig. 4–6). It is important to consider all of the possible causes of such failure, because if the descending aorta is not examined the diagnosis may be missed.

The diagnostic finding in coarctation is narrowing of the descending aorta, causing an obstruction to blood flow and a pressure gradient. In the newborn period the findings may be difficult to identify, because the ductus arteriosus can still be open, leading to almost normal flows and pressure in the descending aorta. Even though there might be a significant obstruction, the pressures can be similar, leading to a lack of measurable gradient.

For this reason it can be difficult or impossible to rule out a coarctation in an asymptomatic infant. Conversely, if there are symptoms such as heart failure or signs such as differential cyanosis of the lower extremities, we should be able to find abnormalities on the echocardiographic examination, such as significant obstruction in the first case or a clear connection between the pulmonary artery and descending aorta via an open ductus in the second.

Similarly, if we do find an obstruction, we may have difficulty assessing the severity while the ductus is still open both because of the reasons noted previously and because the process of ductal closure may cause further obstruction by distorting the anatomy of the descending aorta.

As noted in the next section, a significant percentage of patients with aortic coarctation also have other cardiac defects, most frequently aortic or mitral valve abnormalities or ventricular septal defects.

When You Find One Abnormality, Look for Others

In addition to the expected anomalies with each syndrome, there is another set of associations, which, although not a part of the actual syndrome, can often be found together. A general principle can be stated for all age groups: once you have found an abnormality, the probability of finding another is higher than it was to find the first. If, for example, the general incidence of heart defects is about 1.0%, the chance of finding an abnormality on a "screening" examination in all newborns should be about that value. Once an initial abnormality had been identified, however, the chance of finding another in the same patient would be greater, perhaps 25% to 50%. This can be even higher in the case of defined syndromes but is also true when the patient does not have a known syndrome.

Table 4–4. Frequent Association of Findings

Primary Defect	Associated Defects
Coarctation	Bicuspid aortic valve, mitral valve anomalies, VSD, PDA
Perimembranous VSD	Aortic insufficiency
Supracristal VSD	Aortic insufficiency
Ebstein's anomaly	Atrial septal defect
Transposition	Atrial septal defect, ventricular septal defect

VSD, ventricular septal defect; PDA, patent ductus arteriosus.

As an example, when the patient has a coarctation, we know that more than 50% of those patients have other cardiac defects, which most commonly involve the aortic valve, mitral valve, or ventricular septal defects. This means that we should make special efforts to look for these defects if we identify a coarctation and resist the temptation to "rest on our laurels" when we have identified and characterized the first defect.

There are many such associations, and the accuracy of the echocardiographic examination can be significantly enhanced by an awareness of them. The most common and important associations are listed in Table 4–4.

EFFECTS ON THE HEART OF OTHER DISEASE

The heart plays a major role in many of the problems in the newborn, especially those including respiratory difficulty. For that reason, most of these have already been dealt with in the sections on respiratory problems and cyanosis. In some cases, however, the cardiac problems are secondary but still of clinical significance. These are listed next. Problems that are primarily fetal, such as "foramen ovale closure," are not dealt with here.

Pulmonary Disease

When there is significant pulmonary disease, pulmonary hypertension often results.

This can be evaluated using the tricuspid insufficiency velocity to calculate the right ventricular to right atrial pressure gradient. The normal newborn has a relative right ventricular hypertrophy, and further hypertrophy takes a while to develop, so measurable right ventricular hypertrophy occurs only if the pulmonary problems are long-standing. Finally, there is the issue of the open ductus, which has been discussed in the section on respiratory problems.

Difficult Resuscitation

After a difficult resuscitation, ventricular function can be reduced because of global ischemia. This will usually return to normal if the condition of the infant improves. In most cases, this diagnosis is clear by clinical history, and other possible causes of a dilated ventricle with reduced function are excluded. This means that there is no evidence for outflow obstruction such as aortic stenosis or coarctation and no evidence for endocardial fibroelastosis.

Infection

Infection commonly does not affect the heart directly but causes a high-output state because of fever and vasodilation. In some forms of sepsis, there may be direct toxic injury to the heart, resulting in decreased systolic function. There may also be pericardial effusion with tamponade.

Examination of the Toddler and Child

METHOD OF EXAMINATION

Perhaps more than at any other age, making the patient comfortable is extremely important for the child and the toddler. Spending a small amount of time at the beginning of the examination can lead to much greater time savings in the examination overall and make the examination process much more pleasant for all concerned. Because the issues in this chapter are similar for both the young child and the toddler, the term "young child" will be used in both cases.

Potentially the most difficult examination is that of the young child who has limited verbal skills but is still strong enough to put up a struggle. Some echocardiographic laboratories will routinely sedate such children before examination, and some studies have even suggested that Doppler measurements are more accurate when the patient is sedated.

In my experience, sedation is rarely required when a small amount of time is spent to make the child comfortable and the examination is directed at the key questions being asked for clinical management. On some occasions, a repeat examination was scheduled after the parents had "play-acted" the ultrasound examination. When this strategy was unsuccessful (less than 1 per 1000 examinations), a repeat examination was scheduled with sedation. Studies comparing echocardiographic estimations of pressure gradients to pressures measured at catheterization point out true differences in the pressure gradients. However, the pressure gradients measured at catheterization are in a sedated patient and are presumed to reflect the physiological state of the awake patient. It seems likely that the measurements made in the unsedated patient with Doppler are probably more representative of the normal physiological state, even though such measurements are not entirely equivalent to the body of literature obtained at catheterization.

The key points to making the child comfortable are a gradual, stepwise approach, a soothing manner, and distraction. Children are frightened by the unfamiliar and by sudden changes in particular. It can be frightening for a smaller child to be addressed directly or be approached too closely, especially early in the encounter. It can also be frightening to be undressed immediately. My approach is to begin by speaking to the parent(s) in a calm and unhurried voice while standing 4 to 5 feet away from the child. If the parents are at ease, the child is more likely to be comfortable as well. It is important that the child be aware that the parents are comfortable with the examiner. During this conversation, you can glance briefly at the child, gauging the reaction. If the child reacts by hiding his or her face or hiding behind the parent, you should look away and try again later during the conversation. If there is little reaction, you can try looking for a longer time. Once you are able to look at the child for a prolonged period while still talking to the parent, you can talk directly to the child in a soothing voice and approach gradually.

It is helpful to talk to the child about the examination and even point to the area where the transducer will be placed during the examination. If the child is nervous, it can help to bring a transducer over for the child to touch. If the child is afraid to touch the transducer, you can touch it yourself or have the parent touch the transducer. If the child is nervous enough to have needed these steps, it can be helpful to place the transducer on the back of the child's hand or knee or even foot and then slowly work your way up to the chest, with the child still clothed. You can then go back to placing the transducer on the bare stomach or "on your belly button," again working slowly up to the chest, all without ultrasound gel. In the case of the very nervous child, all of these steps can be demonstrated on a teddy bear or other play animal first or on the parent.

If the child is very nervous, it may be best to perform the examination with the child clothed and even sitting in a parent's lap. Of the two, removing the clothing is the more important, because it gets in the way of the examination, but many children are quite fearful of removing their clothes, perhaps because they fear an injection. Examination sitting in the parent's lap can be quite reassuring to the child and does not significantly hinder the process. The child can be asked directly whether he or she would prefer to sit in a parent's lap as well as about taking off some clothes. If the child does not respond, the parent can be asked.

The ultrasound gel itself can be frightening, especially if it is cold. The child should at least be warned and, if necessary, allowed to touch the gel and even play with a little on his or her hands.

An array of small toys can be very helpful to engage the interest and distract the young child. Squeezable animals seem to be a favorite, especially if they make a sound and are yellow in color. For this reason, I believe that at least one "yellow, squeaky toy" is an essential piece of equipment for every laboratory examining young children.

The question of whether or not to put the electrocardiographic (ECG) monitoring electrodes on can also affect the success of the examination. The ECG can be essential for timing of cardiac events in certain cases. At the same time, some young children find placing the electrodes to be frightening and the presence of the wires constraining. My approach is to dispense with the placement of the electrodes in the young child, unless it is clear that timing information would be a key part of the examination.

All of the standard views can be obtained in children. The ribs are not completely ossi-fied, especially anteriorly, so that the parasternal windows are often more easily obtained than in teenagers and adults (Fig. 5–1). Typically, a 5 MHz transducer can be used for the entire examination.

The survey examination findings are now more like those for adults than for infants. The pressure relationships resemble those in adults; left-sided ventricular pressures exceed right-sided ventricular pressures by a factor of 4 to 5. Also, the cardiac chambers have had a chance to "grow into" these new pressure relationships (Box 5–1).

The most common clinical presentations in this age group are an asymptomatic murmur, chest pain, and fatigue. By this age, virtually all cyanotic defects have already been diagnosed.

BOX 5–1

SURVEY EXAMINATION IN THE CHILD

Two ventricles

Interventricular septum intact

Right ventricle slightly smaller than left

Two atria

Roughly equal in size

Left atrium <1.5 times aortic diameter

Atrioventricular valves

Each into respective ventricle

Tricuspid displaced slightly toward apex

Mild tricuspid insufficiency common

Semilunar valves

Each from respective ventricle

Pulmonic valve anterior

Mild pulmonic insufficiency normal

Great arteries

Pulmonary artery and aorta cross

No evidence for ductal flow

No flow acceleration in aorta or pulmonary arteries

Other

Right ventricular pressure estimate <28 mm Hg

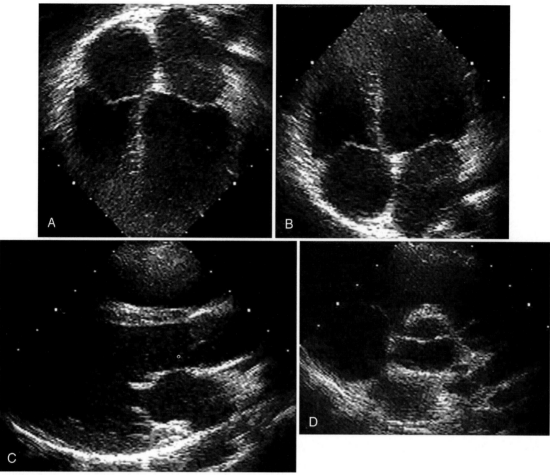

Figure 5–1. *A,* The apical four-chamber view in a normal 11-year-old child in the standard "pediatric" view. *B,* The same image in an "adult" view. Note that the right ventricle is slightly smaller than the left and the tricuspid septal insertion is displaced slightly toward the ventricular apex. These are normal findings. *C,* The parasternal long axis. *D,* The parasternal short axis at the aortic valve level. Note that when the aortic outflow is in cross-section, the right ventricular and pulmonic outflow are imaged lengthwise, demonstrating the crossing of these two structures.

ASYMPTOMATIC MURMUR

Asymptomatic murmurs in school-age children are very common. In the vast majority of cases, there is no associated structural heart disease, and the murmur is called innocent, or functional. The incidence of such functional murmurs is extremely high; it is estimated that as many as 50% of all children have a form of murmur at some time during their childhood. The source of functional murmurs is sometimes questioned, but this is perhaps the wrong focus. Rather, we might ask why we cannot hear the blood flow in all patients. The rea-

son has to do with the limits of our hearing, the velocity of blood flow, and the distance to the structures of interest. Because the distances in the child are smaller, it seems logical that we can hear this flow more often. When confronted with children with an asymptomatic murmur, the challenge is to rule out potential structural disease while reliably identifying normal individuals as such.

A helpful distinction is the patient's type of murmur. The spectrum of possible diagnoses is very different for a systolic versus a diastolic murmur, and a continuous murmur is quite different as well. If this infor-

Table 5–1. Common Diagnostic Possibilities for Asymptomatic Murmur in a Child

Timing	Functional Cause	Pathological Cause
Systolic	Still's "Tricuspid" Subclavian bruit	Ventricular septal defect Aortic stenosis Pulmonic stenosis Atrial septal defect Coarctation
Diastolic	None	Aortic insufficiency Pulmonic insufficiency Mitral stenosis
Continuous	Venous hum	Patent ductus arteriosus Arteriovenous malformation/fistula Ruptured sinus of Valsalva aneurysm

mation is available, it can be extremely helpful in directing the examination because it limits the possibilities (Table 5–1)

What Is Most Likely?

It is most likely that an asymptomatic murmur does not represent disease but rather is a normal variant. There are many different varieties of functional murmurs. Some may have characteristic findings on echocardiographic examination, and others may have none. Because the murmur is the reason for the examination, it is helpful to know what could be related to the murmur.

A systolic functional murmur is most commonly a Still's murmur, which is typically located at the left sternal border and has a "musical" or "humming" quality. This is the most common functional murmur of childhood and usually is noticed between 3 and 6 years of age. The cause is unknown, but there may be an association with "false tendons" or fibromuscular chords that cross the left ventricle. In any case, there is no associated significant structural disease or functional disorder.

A second common type of functional systolic murmur is similar to Still's murmur but is harsher in quality, although still low pitched, and located at the left lower sternal border. The cause of this murmur is likewise unknown but is perhaps related to the func-

tional tricuspid regurgitation found in up to 80% of normal individuals. Clearly, finding tricuspid regurgitation supports this conclusion but is not diagnostic because it is present in many normal individuals.

A third common type of functional systolic murmur is the subclavian bruit. This is a murmur heard supraclavicularly and in the suprasternal notch but is not heard as well at the upper sternal border. This distinguishes it from aortic stenosis. It is believed to be caused by turbulence at the branch point of the subclavian artery, usually the right, which may even be visible on color Doppler examination.

The final common type of functional systolic murmur is the pulmonary flow murmur. In terms of location, it is best heard at the left upper sternal border and typically has a soft, blowing quality. Although it is usually easily distinguished from pulmonic stenosis, which has a much harsher quality, it may be difficult to distinguish, based on quality and location, from the flow murmur found with an atrial septal defect. This distinction should be easily made on echocardiographic examination, as discussed in the next section.

One type of continuous murmur, the venous hum, is functional. This murmur is usually heard best at the right supraclavicular space when the patient is upright, and it varies with respiration. It is probably caused by turbulence in the jugular venous flow. There are no particular echocardiographic findings.

Purely diastolic murmurs are rare and must always be considered as representing disease, although venous hums can sometimes be most prominent in diastole.

What Is Unlikely But Potentially Significant?

With the very high incidence of functional murmurs, finding a real defect is improbable. Most of the significant defects present during infancy, but there are conditions that can appear later in life, or there may be defects that were missed for one reason or another. As mentioned, diastolic murmurs should be considered pathological until proven otherwise. The most common causes of a diastolic murmur are aortic and pulmonic insufficiency, although atrioventricular valve stenosis sometimes causes audible diastolic murmurs. The most likely causes of a pathological asymptomatic systolic murmur in a child are presented in Box 5–2.

Ventricular Septal Defect

Although most ventricular septal defects are detected in infancy, occasionally a defect is missed early on and only detected in childhood. There can be many reasons for this. As mentioned in Chapter 2, at birth the pressures in the pulmonary circulation are high and the degree of left-to-right shunting is correspondingly low. The lack of a significant pressure gradient reduces the amplitude and pitch of the sound produced by the shunt, in some cases so much so that it is completely inaudible at birth. It is usually easier to diagnose a ventricular septal defect some days after birth, both by auscultation and echocardiographic examination. A defect in an older infant may go undetected if he or she was fussy at presentation, preventing adequate examination.

Of the types of ventricular septal defects that might be present, the most likely would be a perimembranous defect or a muscular defect, and it is also highly probable that the defect is restrictive (i.e., has a significant pressure gradient and a small shunt) (Figs. 5–2 and 5–3; see also color figures). If it were not restrictive, the probability is high that the child would have had congestive heart failure as an infant, and the defect would have been discovered. The exception is when there is a restriction of flow to

the lungs as a result of pulmonic stenosis, peripheral pulmonic stenosis, or increased pulmonary vascular resistance. In the first two cases, the murmur is usually loud enough to prompt evaluation and diagnosis at an early age, whereas the latter is usually accompanied by significant problems with oxygenation, which would also lead to an early evaluation. Conversely, if the right-sided pressures are elevated, it is much easier to miss a concomitant ventricular septal defect because the pressure difference is lower, and flow across the defect would not be as disturbed.

Finding a small ventricular septal defect may require a thorough search because the range of locations is wide. One tip is that the point at which the murmur is loudest is often the location where the jet is pointed and, therefore, the point at which the Doppler signal is maximal. Thus, a few moments using a stethoscope to locate the point at which the murmur is loudest and placing the ultrasound transducer there first can often help narrow the search, saving time.

In addition, when looking for a ventricular septal defect, color Doppler imaging is especially good for screening large areas, although there is the possibility of false-positive results. Any findings with color Doppler should be confirmed with high-pulse-repetition-frequency (HPRF) or continuous-wave (CW) Doppler (Box 5–3 and Fig. 5–4; see also color figure).

In spite of this uncertainty, a ventricular septal defect detected in childhood is most likely found in one of three locations. The first is the perimembranous position. The best transducer location to find such a ventricular septal defect is from the left (or sometimes right) parasternal window in the second or third intercostal space, using the long-axis or short-axis orientation. Usually the flow from the defect is most easily detected with CW Doppler, although other Doppler techniques can be used as well. Because of the low frame rate, color Doppler can sometimes yield an apparent false-positive result because of tricuspid inflow, which is picked up by the side lobes of the beam. Similarly, small areas of disturbed flow can emulate a ventricular septal defect as well.

BOX 5–2
MOST COMMON CAUSES OF PATHOLOGICAL SYSTOLIC MURMURS IN THE CHILD

Ventricular septal defect

Atrial septal defect

Aortic stenosis

Pulmonic stenosis

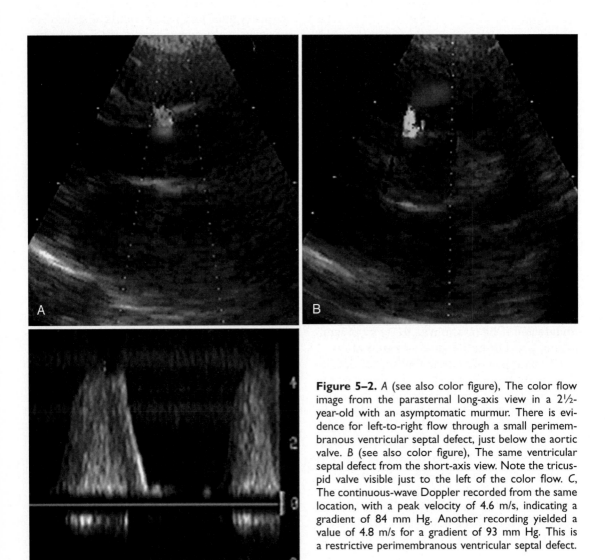

Figure 5–2. *A* (see also color figure), The color flow image from the parasternal long-axis view in a 2½-year-old with an asymptomatic murmur. There is evidence for left-to-right flow through a small perimembranous ventricular septal defect, just below the aortic valve. *B* (see also color figure), The same ventricular septal defect from the short-axis view. Note the tricuspid valve visible just to the left of the color flow. *C*, The continuous-wave Doppler recorded from the same location, with a peak velocity of 4.6 m/s, indicating a gradient of 84 mm Hg. Another recording yielded a value of 4.8 m/s for a gradient of 93 mm Hg. This is a restrictive perimembranous ventricular septal defect.

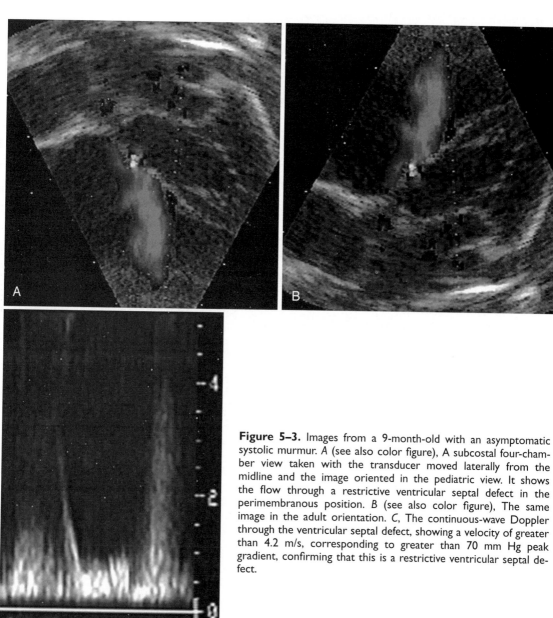

Figure 5–3. Images from a 9-month-old with an asymptomatic systolic murmur. *A* (see also color figure), A subcostal four-chamber view taken with the transducer moved laterally from the midline and the image oriented in the pediatric view. It shows the flow through a restrictive ventricular septal defect in the perimembranous position. *B* (see also color figure), The same image in the adult orientation. *C*, The continuous-wave Doppler through the ventricular septal defect, showing a velocity of greater than 4.2 m/s, corresponding to greater than 70 mm Hg peak gradient, confirming that this is a restrictive ventricular septal defect.

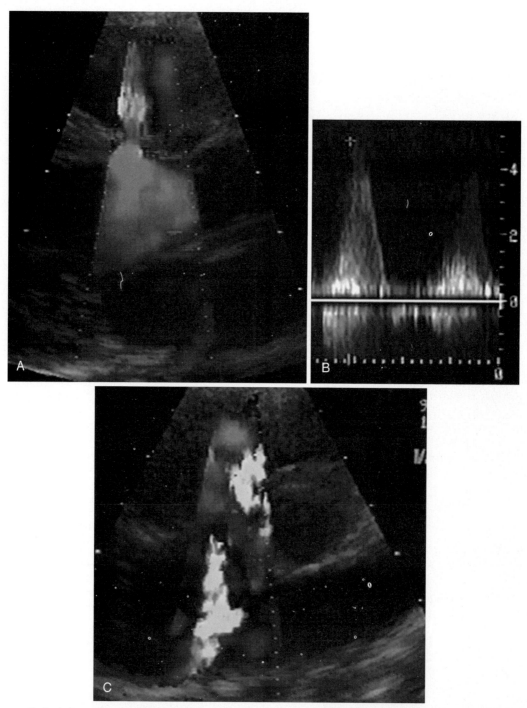

Figure 5–4. *A* (see also color figure), The parasternal long-axis view of the heart of a 13-month-old with an asymptomatic systolic murmur. There is flow from the left ventricle to the right ventricle across a perimembranous ventricular septal defect. Note that this image does not show disturbed flow, which raises the question of elevation of the right-sided pressures, or a false-positive color flow image. *B,* Continuous-wave Doppler shows that the peak velocity is 4.8 m/s, indicating that this is a ventricular septal defect and that there is a gradient of 93 mm Hg. *C* (see also color figure), The short-axis parasternal view, with the relationship of the ventricular septal defect flow and the tricuspid regurgitation.

BOX 5–3
TIPS FOR DIAGNOSIS OF
VENTRICULAR SEPTAL DEFECTS

Place Doppler transducer where the
murmur is loudest.

Do not forget the low parasternal and
subcostal views.

Confirm all color Doppler findings with
continuous wave or high-pulse-repetition-
frequency Doppler.

Beware the situation in which the right
ventricular pressure is elevated.

Color Doppler in the short-axis view can be extremely helpful in distinguishing a perimembranous defect from a supracristal defect, however, because the locations are quite distinct on this view.

Small muscular defects can occur anywhere in the muscular septum (see Fig. 4–21) but tend to be in one of two locations. One is at the apex of the right ventricular cavity. These defects often cause a murmur that is best heard at the apex of the heart, and the abnormal flow is often detected best with the transducer at the apical or subcostal position. This type of defect is often missed when only the more "standard" views are used. The other typical location for a small muscular defect is anteriorly, at the junction of the interventricular septum and the right ventricular free wall. This type of defect is often best detected on parasternal views but frequently from a lower interspace than perimembranous defects (i.e., from the third or fourth intercostal space).

Another type of ventricular septal defect that may be associated with a murmur, but of a completely different type, is the atrioventricular septal defect. As mentioned in Chapter 2, these consist of a constellation of abnormalities, which always includes a cleft mitral valve. Mitral insufficiency from this cleft may be the cause of the murmur that is best heard. The diagnosis is made by noting the cleft in the anterior mitral valve leaflet or more often by showing that the mitral and tricuspid valves are at the same level, instead of having the tricuspid valve closer to the ventricular apex. Whenever this defect is diagnosed, one should look for a primum atrial septal defect and the typical ventricular septal defect between the atrioventricular valves (see Fig. 4–24). For the full assessment of an atrioventricular septal defect, the degree of mitral regurgitation should be evaluated as well as the detailed anatomy of the leaflets of the mitral and tricuspid valve. The location of the insertion of the chordae of the anterior mitral valve leaflet has a significant effect on the difficulty of repair.

For all of these ventricular septal defects, after making the diagnosis, a key part of the evaluation is to determine the physiological consequences. Estimation of the right ventricular pressure through measurement of the peak velocity of tricuspid regurgitation and pulmonic insufficiency is very important, as is the estimation of the interventricular gradient by measuring the peak velocity across the ventricular defect. If the defect is a very small muscular defect, the CW signal may be truncated as a result of closure of the defect during systole, and the peak velocities may be alarmingly low, suggesting pulmonary hypertension. In this case, more weight should be placed on tricuspid insufficiency and pulmonic insufficiency. If the right ventricular pressure is high and there is no pulmonic stenosis, the patient is automatically in a higher risk category than if the right ventricular pressure is normal. Other features that should be checked are left atrial size (increased if there is a large shunt), left ventricular size (also increased in large shunts), presence of aortic insufficiency, and other commonly associated defects (Box 5–4).

As mentioned in Chapter 2, aortic insufficiency is highly associated with supracristal ventricular septal defects, occurring in 5% to 7% of patients with this type of lesion. It is also associated with perimembranous ventricular septal defects in 2% to 5% of patients with this lesion.

Atrial Septal Defect

Probably the defects most likely to go undetected for many years are secundum

---

BOX 5–4

POTENTIAL FINDINGS IN VENTRICULAR SEPTAL DEFECT IN AN ASYMPTOMATIC CHILD

Ventricles

  Disturbed flow in region of interventricular septum

Atria

  Left atrial enlargement

Atrioventricular valves

  Tricuspid at same level as mitral

  Cleft mitral valve

  Mitral regurgitation

Semilunar valves

  Aortic insufficiency

Great arteries

  Coarctation

Other

  Elevation of right ventricular pressure

---

atrial septal defects and the physiologically similar partial anomalous pulmonary veins. Either of these can remain undetected for decades but may be discovered during childhood as a result of a flow murmur or large heart on chest x-ray film. Patients with one of these conditions usually do not have a prominent murmur, which is why they can go undetected for so long. If a murmur is present, it is usually a soft, blowing systolic murmur at the left upper sternal border caused by increased pulmonary flow and very similar to the functional pulmonary flow murmur. For these reasons, echocardiography can be helpful in making the diagnosis, which can otherwise be difficult (Fig. 5–5; see also color figure).

The main finding on echocardiography of a patient with a left-to-right shunt at the atrial level is enlargement of the right-sided chambers (Box 5–5). This is due to the volume load caused by the excess flow through the pulmonary circulation. This is usually best assessed from the apical four-chamber view and the parasternal short-axis views. In the apical four-chamber view, the right ventricle is normally not as wide as the left ventricle. Parasternally, it is more difficult to create a standard, so experience is necessary.

The significant volume load to the right ventricle causes several other abnormalities that we can use to confirm the physiology. The increased volume load of the right ventricle caused by the left-to-right shunt is predominantly a diastolic load. This causes distention of the right ventricle and a shift of the interventricular septum toward the left ventricle during diastole. This gives the characteristic D-shaped left ventricle in the short-axis views. During systole, the greater pressure in the left ventricle causes the interventricular septum to bow in the normal direction toward the right ventricle. This motion of the interventricular septum is the opposite of the normal systolic motion and is, therefore, termed "paradoxical." These findings are best appreciated from the parasternal views, and M-mode is particularly helpful in demonstrating the paradoxical septal motion (Figs. 5–5 and 5–6; see also color figure).

Direct visualization of the atrial septal defect is often possible. The best views are from the subcostal approach because the ultrasound beam is perpendicular to the atrial septum, allowing best visualization of the

---

BOX 5–5

POTENTIAL FINDINGS IN ATRIAL LEVEL SHUNTS (ATRIAL SEPTAL DEFECTS AND PARTIAL ANOMALOUS PULMONARY VEINS)

Ventricles

  Enlarged right ventricle

  D-shaped left ventricle

  "Paradoxical" septal motion

Atria

  Right atrial enlargement

  Flow across interatrial septum

Atrioventricular and semilunar valves

  Evidence for increased right-sided flows

Other

  Elevated right ventricular and pulmonary artery pressures

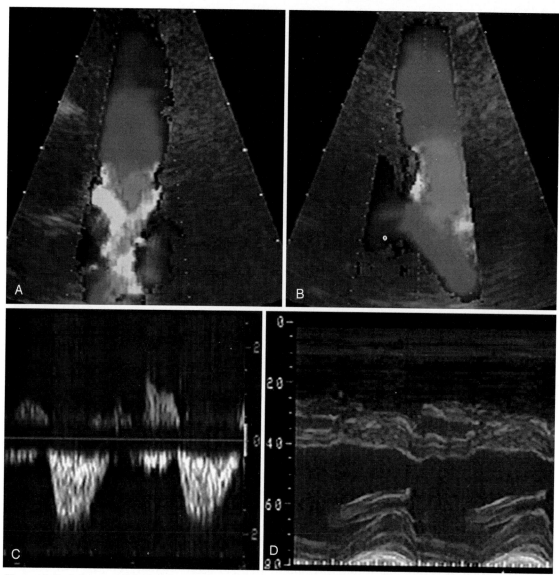

Figure 5–5. A 5-year-old child with a pulmonary systolic murmur. *A* (see also color figure), The color flow through the pulmonary outflow from the parasternal short-axis view. Note the disturbed (green) flow. This could be pulmonic stenosis or atrial septal defect or a normal variant. *B* (see also color figure), At other times in the cardiac cycle, the flow is not disturbed but does exceed the velocity-aliasing limit, changing color to red. *C*, The continuous-wave Doppler recording of this pulmonary flow, demonstrating that the peak velocity is less than 2 m/s, so there is no significant stenosis. *D*, The M-mode of the left ventricle and interventricular septum, showing that there is paradoxical septal motion.

Illustration continued on following page

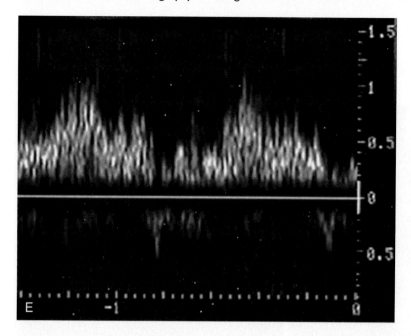

Figure 5–5 *Continued. E,* The Doppler recording of the flow through the atrial septal defect.

septum without dropout. Although many examiners use the apical views, these should be interpreted with caution because there can often be dropout as a result of the atrial septum being parallel to the ultrasound beam. This can lead to a false-positive diagnosis of atrial septal defect.

Color flow can identify flow across the atrial septum, but one should also be careful about this finding. Because of the side lobes of the ultrasound beam, from the subcostal view it is possible to see flow appearing to cross the interatrial septum, although it is actually normal flow from the superior vena cava. There are two ways to avoid this misinterpretation. The first is to angle the plane of the transducer anteriorly to image the superior vena cava flow directly. By keeping the transducer orientation otherwise the same, it is possible to identify the superior vena cava as the source of flow if it originates from the same direction. If the two flows are clearly distinguishable as to direction, it is less likely that this represents a side lobe artifact. The second is to observe the respiratory variation of flow. When the patient breathes in, the intrathoracic pressure is reduced, and venous return through the superior vena cava is increased. During exhalation, there is an increase in the intrathoracic pressure, which leads to a decrease in venous return. These changes

are reflected in an increased velocity of superior vena cava flow (and inferior vena cava flow) during inspiration and, conversely, a decreased velocity during expiration.

Exactly the opposite occurs with the flow across an atrial septal defect. Because of the increased venous return through the venae cavae during inspiration, there is an increase in atrial distension and, therefore, an increase in pressure relative to the left atrium. Because the interatrial gradient is diminished, the flow velocity across the atrial septum decreases. Exactly the opposite occurs during expiration, with a resulting increase in flow. Thus, the respiratory variation of flow across the interatrial septum is exactly opposite that of the superior vena cava, and this allows for distinction between the two (see Fig. 6–3).

Another window that often allows for good imaging of an atrial septal defect is the parasternal short axis. The atrial septum itself as well as the transseptal flow can be well visualized in many patients. The respiratory changes in flow can also be measured from this window.

From the apical window, flow from the inferior vena cava can be directed toward the interatrial septum, swirling away from the septum as it enters the atrium. This may give an appearance similar to an atrial

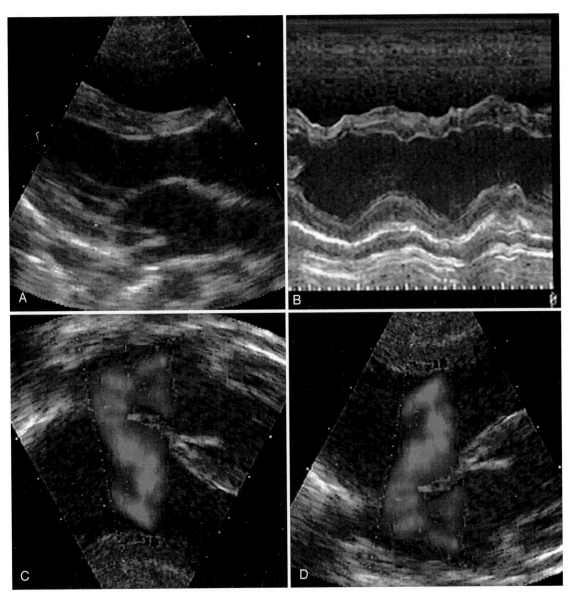

Figure 5–6. A 9-month-old with a pulmonary flow murmur. A, The long-axis parasternal view. Note how the right ventricle appears slightly larger than normal, and the interventricular septum bows toward the left ventricle. B, The M-mode of the left ventricle and interventricular septum, showing how the septum moves posteriorly during diastole and anteriorly during early systole (when thickening) compared with the posterior wall, which moves normally. This is termed paradoxical septal motion and is indicative of right ventricular volume overload. C and D (see also color figure), The subcostal four-chamber view in the standard pediatric and adult orientations, respectively, demonstrating color flow across the interatrial septum, from the left atrium to right atrium.

septal defect flow (Fig. 5–7; see also color figure). The same maneuvers just mentioned to distinguish superior vena cava flow can be used to reduce the risk of misdiagnosis, but one should not rely on the apical view for the diagnosis of atrial septal defects.

If physiological changes of a large volume load on the right side are present but no atrial septal defect is visualized, several possibilities can be considered (Box 5–6). The first is insufficiency of the tricuspid or pulmonic valves. This will cause all of the signs of volume loading on the right side of the heart, but there is no shunt. Another possibility is a sinus venosus defect. The location of this type of defect is difficult to visualize and may require transesophageal imaging for confirmation. The final possibility is partial anomalous pulmonary veins, which can also be associated with secundum atrial septal defects and sinus venosus defects. It is rare that these can be visualized directly, but they should be suspected whenever there are signs of right ventricular volume load but no evidence for an atrial septal defect or significant insufficiency of the pulmonic or tricuspid valves.

If we detect a shunt, we should always assess the physiological consequences. The most serious is elevation of the pulmonary artery pressure, which we can assess from the velocity of tricuspid insufficiency or pulmonic insufficiency. If this pressure is elevated, we should recall that it can be due to increases in flow as well as vascular resistance. For this reason, it is especially important to assess relative flow when right-sided pressures are elevated. This can be done using the continuity equation as discussed in Chapter 1. It is possible that the increase in pressure is entirely due to increased flow, with no increase in vascular resistance. In this case, the prognosis is better than when there is normal flow and increased pressures are due entirely to increased vascular resistance.

Aortic Stenosis

An important but fortunately infrequent cause of murmur in children is aortic stenosis. As was noted in Chapter 2, this can be located at one of three different levels: subvalvular, valvular, or supravalvular. The echocardiographic appearance is quite different, although the evaluation of the physiological consequences is similar.

Subvalvular stenosis comes in two varieties: membranous and muscular. The membranous type consists of a fibrous ring below the aortic valve in the left ventricular outflow tract. This ring can consist of a thin membrane, which can be difficult to visualize on two-dimensional imaging, or it can be a thicker band or even occasionally a tubular narrowing, both of which are more visible on imaging. The parasternal and apical views are usually best for imaging and apical views best for CW Doppler examination. In all cases, there will be disturbed flow on color Doppler examination, originating at the site of the narrowing, and a velocity increase with CW or HPRF Doppler. In both of these varieties of membranous subvalvular aortic stenosis, there can be an associated aortic insufficiency, which should be looked for and evaluated.

The muscular form of outflow obstruction is less common but of great importance if present, because it is one of the main causes of sudden death in athletes. Muscular outflow obstruction develops over time in those who are predisposed to it. This predisposition can be sporadic or familial. On two-dimensional examination, there is usually an asymmetric thickening of the interventricular septum, so that it bulges into the left ventricular outflow tract (Fig. 5–8). The obstruction is dynamic, which means that it varies both during the cardiac cycle and

---

BOX 5–6
CAUSES OF RIGHT VENTRICULAR
VOLUME OVERLOAD (ACYANOTIC)

Shunts
  Atrial septal defects
  Partial anomalous pulmonary veins
Regurgitation
  Tricuspid insufficiency
  Pulmonic insufficiency

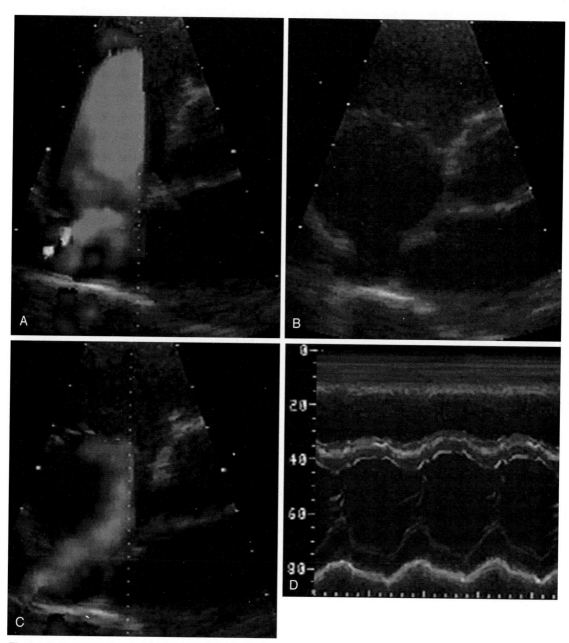

Figure 5–7. Images from a 6-year-old with an asymptomatic murmur. *A* (see also color figure), The parasternal short-axis view of the atrial septum with color looks like a secundum atrial septal defect. In fact, this is flow from the inferior vena cava. *B,* With tissue imaging alone, it is evident how the eustachian valve gives the appearance of a rim of atrial septum, and the true septum is almost parallel to the ultrasound beam and, therefore, not as visible. *C* (see also color figure), A slight change in angle shows the flow coming from the inferior vena cava. The M-mode *(D)* showed no evidence for paradoxical septal motion, although this can be absent in some patients with atrial septal defects.

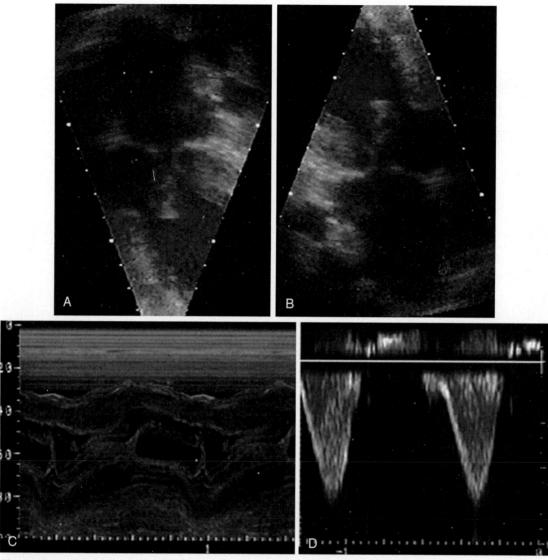

Figure 5–8. Images from a 12-year-old girl with dyspnea and chest pain on exertion. *A* and *B*, The same view in the pediatric and adult orientations, respectively. This is an apical long-axis view, showing the left ventricle and left ventricular outflow tract. There is hypertrophy of the left ventricle and systolic anterior motion of the anterior leaflet of the mitral valve. *C*, The same findings on M-mode. *D*, The high-pulse-repetition-frequency Doppler recording through the area of maximal velocity, with a peak velocity of 4.6 m/s, corresponding to an 85-mm Hg gradient. Note also how the gradient is late peaking, as is typical for a dynamic muscular obstruction rather than a static obstruction. This patient has hypertrophic obstructive cardiomyopathy.

with ventricular loading conditions. This has two consequences. First, the velocity gradient increases during the cardiac cycle, often reaching a peak near the end. This can cause a triangular or "dagger-shaped" waveform, which is typical for this condition. Second, the degree of obstruction can vary on different examinations or even with maneuvers during the examination. For this reason, the dynamic obstruction pattern

should always be noted, even if the gradient seems less than critical.

Valvular aortic stenosis is characterized by doming or decreased opening of the aortic valve on two-dimensional examination (Fig. 5–9) and a velocity increase on CW or HPRF Doppler (Fig. 5–10). Color Doppler shows disturbed flow at the level of the valve. Associated aortic insufficiency is common and should also be evaluated. It is important to

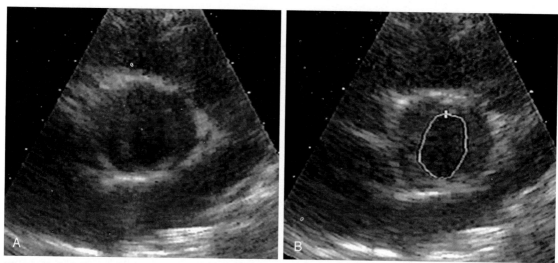

Figure 5–9. *A,* The short-axis view of the aortic valve in a 12-year-old with a murmur. The aortic valve is bicuspid, with an oval vertical opening. It is possible to measure the area of the opening, as has been done in *B* on the same patient. This valve had an opening of 2.1 cm², so the degree of stenosis must be graded as mild.

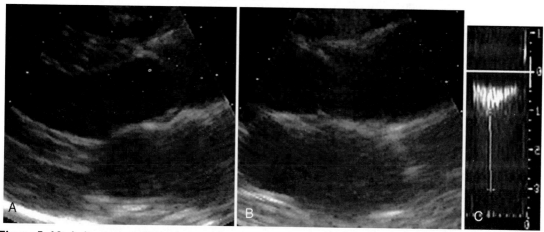

Figure 5–10. *A,* A parasternal long-axis view from an 11-year-old child with a murmur. Of note is that aortic valve leaflets do not open fully, displaying a "domed" pattern during systole, which is when this image was recorded. This is due to congenital aortic stenosis. *B,* Shows the ascending aorta above the valve, with evidence of poststenotic dilatation. *C,* Continuous-wave Doppler through the valve, recorded from the apical window. It is possible to see the low-velocity flow in the left ventricular outflow tract as well as the high-velocity flow through the stenotic valve. The cursors are at the peak velocity for both, which were 1.0 and 3.0 m/s, respectively. This yields a peak gradient of (36 − 4 = 32 mm Hg). Therefore, the hemodynamic severity of this aortic stenosis is mild at this time.

define the structure of the valve and the number of cusps it has. This is best done in the parasternal short-axis views. If the valve has three cusps and the stenosis is due to some commissural fusion, there is a possibility of repair. Repair is unlikely if the valve is bicuspid or unicuspid, although the probability of finding a unicuspid valve in childhood is low.

Supravalvular aortic stenosis is rare and is usually associated with Williams syndrome. The site of the stenosis should be visible on two-dimensional examination from the parasternal views. Evaluation of the physiology is the same as for other forms of aortic stenosis.

In all cases of aortic stenosis, one should also be alert to the association with coarctation of the aorta. This is strongest with bicuspid aortic valve but may be associated with any of the types of aortic stenosis. In some cases, the murmur of mild aortic stenosis may be the reason for referral, but the patient's more serious problem is an aortic coarctation. The best views for detecting a coarctation are from the suprasternal notch. In some cases, the coarctation can be seen on two-dimensional imaging, or the disturbed flow can be detected on color Doppler. However, the best way to detect a coarctation is always CW Doppler from the suprasternal notch.

Pulmonic Stenosis

Pulmonic stenosis, usually with a very mild gradient, is a frequent cause of pathological murmurs found later in childhood in asymptomatic patients. The best transducer position for identifying pulmonic stenosis is usually the parasternal; the highest velocity gradient is most commonly acquired from the right parasternal location. In some cases, the subcostal short axis view is also helpful.

The physiological evaluation is very important for determining the need for treatment, as in many other cases. The right ventricular pressure can be assessed by measuring the gradient across the pulmonic valve and the velocity of tricuspid regurgitation.

Two special cases deserve additional at-tention. The first is infundibular stenosis, which rarely presents in the older child. It is a muscular, subpulmonary narrowing that can occur by itself but is often associated with a ventricular septal defect or some valvular stenosis. Infundibular stenosis is identified by the narrowing of the infundibulum (right ventricular outflow tract) on two-dimensional examination, disturbed flow on color Doppler, and high velocities detected in the infundibulum. Its combination with a ventricular septal defect should be distinguished from tetralogy of Fallot, because the prognosis after repair is thought to be better.

The second is peripheral pulmonic stenosis. In this case the structural examination of the heart is normal, but there might be right ventricular hypertrophy if the degree of stenosis is severe. The site of the stenosis is usually distal enough to be not visible because of lung shadowing. However, if the narrowing is significant, the right ventricular pressure will be elevated, which can be detected by examining the velocity of tricuspid insufficiency. This diagnosis should be suspected when there is an increase in right ventricular systolic pressure in a patient with no obvious stenosis, no shunt lesion identified, and no evidence of lung disease.

Patent Ductus Arteriosus

The most common cause of a pathological continuous murmur in childhood is a persistent ductus arteriosus, usually called a patent ductus arteriosus. Older patients with patent ductus arteriosus are usually asymptomatic with a continuous murmur. Although the physical examination is usually quite characteristic, echocardiography can be used to confirm the diagnosis and rule out potential alternative causes for the murmur.

The flow of a ductus arteriosus from the descending aorta to the pulmonary artery is best detected from the left parasternal location in the short-axis view, using color Doppler (see Chapter 4, Figs. 4–7 to 4–12). CW and HPRF Doppler should always be used to confirm the findings as well as to measure the peak velocity for determination of the pressure difference. If there is no evidence for a patent ductus arteriosus, one should consider alternative pathological causes of a continuous murmur, including a coronary fistula, arteriopulmonary window, and ruptured sinus of Valsalva aneurysm, all of which are discussed further under Chest Pain in this chapter and Chapter 6.

What Is a Sufficient Examination to Rule Out a Cardiac Defect?

The range of defects presented is not exhaustive but merely mentions the more common potential diagnoses. At what point can we determine that our examination was sufficient to rule out a significant cardiac defect?

Understanding that it is impossible to completely rule out a cardiac defect, we can, however, in virtually all cases rule out the possibility of a defect that causes the presenting problem (murmur) or rule out significant cardiac disease.

With this in mind, we can create a type of survey of cardiac structure to rule out significant disease (Box 5–7), consisting of the following:

Normal chamber size: a significant shunt, especially left to right, or significant valvular regurgitation should cause an increase in chamber size.

Slight offset of tricuspid and mitral valves: this would rule out endocardial cushion defects and Ebstein's anomaly (Fig. 5–11; see also color figure).

No evidence of increased velocities in the aortic or pulmonic outflows: this would rule out significant stenosis of these valves.

Normal right ventricular systolic pressure: this avoids the problem of missing a left-to-right shunt resulting from equalization of pressures in the two ventricles and rules out pulmonary hypertension and peripheral pulmonic stenosis.

No evidence for ventricular septal defects: these defects can be a cause of short systolic murmurs.

No evidence for a patent ductus arteriosus: this can be a cause of continuous murmur.

No evidence for an aortic coarctation: this

BOX 5–7
SUFFICIENT EXAMINATION TO RULE OUT A PATHOLOGICAL CARDIAC CAUSE OF MURMUR

Ventricles
  Right slightly smaller than left
  No disturbed flow across ventricular septum
Atria
  Equal and normal in size
  No flow across interatrial septum
Atrioventricular valves
  Tricuspid closer to apex than mitral by a small amount
  No significant regurgitation
Semilunar valves
  No evidence for stenosis
  No evidence for regurgitation of aortic valve
  No evidence for significant regurgitation of pulmonic valve
Great arteries
  No evidence for coarctation
  No evidence for ductus arteriosus
Other
  No evidence for elevation of right ventricular systolic pressures

---

must be examined from the suprasternal notch.

No evidence for significant valvular regurgitation: regurgitation of the tricuspid, pulmonic, and mitral valves can be present in trace to mild quantities in normal individuals. Aortic regurgitation is always an abnormal finding (Fig. 5–12; see also color figure). Tricuspid and mitral insufficiency may cause systolic murmurs, and pulmonic and aortic regurgitation can cause diastolic murmurs.

CHEST PAIN AND FATIGUE

Chest pain and fatigue are fairly frequent complaints among older children and adolescents. Fortunately, the cause is seldom

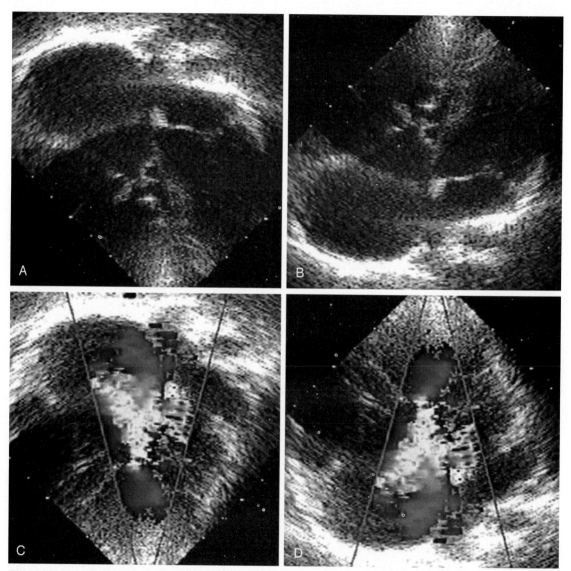

Figure 5–11. *A* and *B*, The apical four-chamber view of a 9-year-old with a murmur and atrial arrhythmias, in the standard pediatric and adult orientations, respectively. Note the significant dilatation of the right side of the heart and the displacement of the tricuspid valve toward the apex, making the diagnosis of Ebstein's anomaly. *C* and *D* (see also color figure), The standard pediatric and adult orientations of an off-axis four-chamber view of the same child, demonstrating significant color flow coming from a left ventricular to right atrial shunt. Note that the tricuspid valve to the left of the color sector is not the source of all of the disturbed flow.

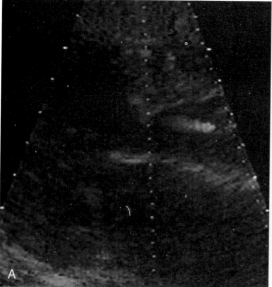
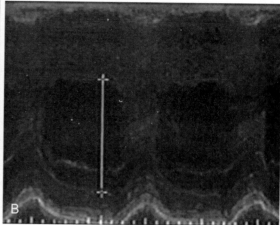

Figure 5–12. *A* (see also color figure), The color Doppler of aortic insufficiency in an 18-year-old who has an asymptomatic diastolic murmur. The view is a parasternal long axis, and a small jet of aortic insufficiency is visible. *B,* The M-mode of the same child's left ventricle with an end-diastolic dimension of 53.5 mm, showing that there is no significant enlargement.

cardiac and usually not even pathological, but cardiac causes are always serious if present. For this reason, we must have a strategy for identifying cardiac causes, if present.

As in previous sections, our approach is "divide and conquer." We can identify the potential cardiac causes of chest pain or fatigue and, therefore, can also identify the findings that must be present for each of these causes. We can then use the echocardiogram to look for these findings. If none is present, we have ruled out a cardiac cause of the symptom.

What Are Potential Cardiac Causes?

The cardiac reasons for chest pain and fatigue in the child are very similar to those in the adult. An example is chest pain resulting from ischemia. The causes of chest pain are often different, however, and much more rare than in adults; atherosclerotic coronary artery disease is extremely rare, and instead congenital coronary anomalies or Kawasaki's induced coronary disease can be found (Box 5–8).

Chest Pain

Most instances of cardiac chest pain are caused by a mismatch between the energy demand of the heart and its blood supply. Ischemic heart disease is the classic example of this in the adult, although it is usually due to acquired heart disease rather than a congenital defect. There is a limita-

---

BOX 5–8
PATHOLOGICAL CAUSES OF CHEST PAIN IN THE CHILD

Congenital coronary anomalies

  Anomalous coronary origin

  Coronary fistula

Acquired coronary disease

  Kawasaki's disease

  Emboli

Aortic stenosis

Hypertrophic cardiomyopathy

Dilated cardiomyopathy

Pericarditis

Sinus of Valsalva aneurysm rupture

tion of the blood supply to the heart because of a narrowing of the coronary arteries. When demand is increased by exercise, chest pain (angina pectoris) results.

Although ischemic disease of this classic variety can occur in children rarely, when resulting from progeria or hyperlipidemic disorders, other forms of mismatch are more common (Table 5–2). These can be subdivided into those caused by either decreased supply or increased demand.

In order for there to be a decreased supply, there must be a disorder of the coronary arteries. This can be either congenital or acquired. The congenital variety of coronary anomaly is extremely variable; one or more coronary arteries have either an anomalous origin in the pulmonary artery or an origin in the aorta and an abnormal course. When one or more coronary arteries originates in the pulmonary artery, the direction of blood flow is reversed, because there are usually collaterals connecting the coronary vessels, and the other vessels will be connected to the aorta, which has a much higher pressure. The result is that the blood flow through the normal vessels will be greatly increased, and these vessels may be dilated. Blood flow in the anomalous vessel will be from the collaterals toward the pulmonary artery. The pressure in the anomalous vessel will be much lower than normal. As a result, the perfusion pressure of the area of myocardium supplied by that vessel will be quite low. This is the area that can have

Table 5–2. Potential Findings in Pathological Chest Pain in the Child

Cause	Findings
Coronary disease	Segmental wall motion abnormalities Abnormal origin of coronary arteries Thickening of coronary arteries
Aortic stenosis	Abnormal valve motion Increased velocity through valve
Cardiomyopathy	Dilated left ventricle Thickened ventricular walls Decreased systolic function
Other	Sinus of Valsalva aneurysm with rupture Pericardial thickening/fluid

abnormal function, even at rest, and may be a source for chest pain with exertion. The other type of coronary anomaly is an abnormal course for an artery originating in the aorta. The abnormal artery may pass between the aorta and pulmonary artery, which can lead to compression, especially during exercise.

Anomalous coronary arteries that cause symptoms will usually result in wall function abnormalities, usually termed "wall motion abnormalities." In fact, it may be misleading to look at wall motion alone, because we can be fooled by a translation motion of the heart. It is more accurate to examine wall thickening as an assessment of wall function.

Surprisingly often, it is possible to actually see the anomalous vessels on the two-dimensional examination as well as measure the abnormal direction and pattern of flow with Doppler. This is because the increased blood flow in such vessels leads to dilation, and both the dilation and increased flow make visualization easier.

Coronary aneurysm is the most common form of acquired coronary artery disease in children secondary to Kawasaki's disease. These aneurysms may grow quite large and can form thrombi, which can then cause ischemia from either occlusion or embolization. These aneurysms occur long after the initial illness and may be visible on echocardiographic examination of the coronaries from the parasternal short-axis view. Although the aneurysms are frequently detectable in the first few centimeters of the coronary arteries visible on echocardiographic examination, not seeing any abnormality in the limited obtainable views of the coronaries possible cannot positively rule out Kawasaki's coronary artery disease. An earlier stage of the pathological changes of Kawasaki's disease is thickening of the wall of the coronary arteries, which may be difficult to identify.

Ischemic chest pain resulting from increased demand may occur in a number of conditions in children. Any condition that raises the pressure in the ventricles will increase myocardial oxygen demand, including aortic stenosis, hypertrophic cardiomyopathy, pulmonary hypertension, and severe

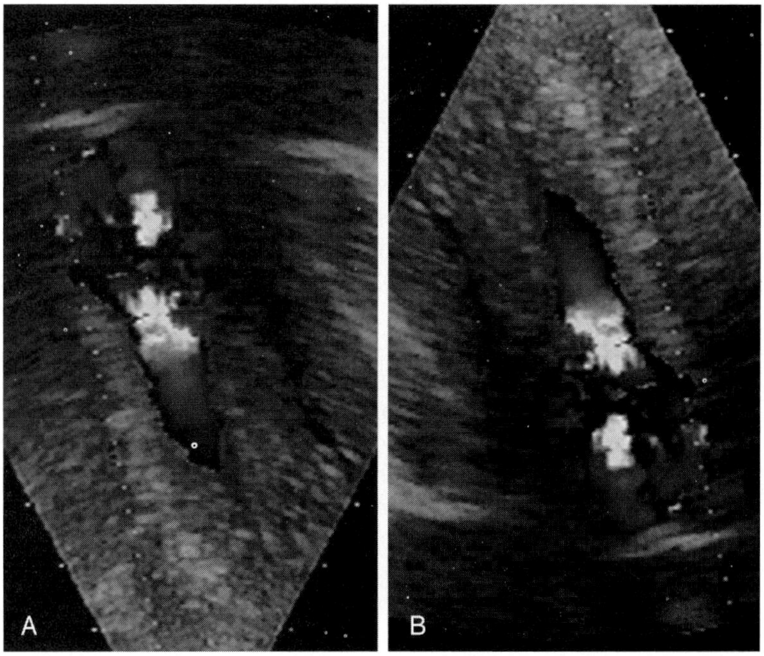

Figure 5–13. These color images are from the same child as in Figure 5–8 and are the same image, shown in different orientations. *A* (see also color figure), The pediatric orientation. *B* (see also color figure), The adult orientation. Each is a color Doppler of the left ventricular outflow tract taken from the apical position. Note the disturbed flow in the left ventricular outflow tract, due to the muscular obstruction.

pulmonic stenosis, to name a few. In aortic stenosis and hypertrophic cardiomyopathy, there can also be a limitation of perfusion pressure of the coronary arteries during exercise, causing a reduction in supply as well.

Cardiomyopathies of both the dilated and hypertrophic varieties can occasionally cause chest pain. This is easy to understand in the case of an obstructive hypertrophic cardiomyopathy (Fig. 5–13; see also color figure), which will increase demand while limiting supply, much like aortic stenosis. It is more difficult to understand for dilated cardiomyopathies, because it seems that supply is not limited. This is not quite true, however. Most of coronary blood flow to the left ventricle occurs during diastole because of the high left ventricular pressures during systole. The intramural wall pressure of the left ventricle during diastole is a function of the left ventricular diastolic pressure and left ventricular dimensions. For the same pressure, the intramural pressure will be higher if the dimensions are larger. In dilated cardiomyopathy, both are increased, so that diastolic intramural pressure is quite elevated, causing an obstruction to the diastolic blood flow. Even though this is a reasonable scenario for ischemic pain in cardiomyopathies, it is not clear whether this is the actual cause of the pain.

The prior discussion has been directed at chronic pain syndromes. Occasionally, children will present with acute chest pain, and this has a distinctly different differential diagnosis list. In these cases, we should consider myocardial infarction (rare) or rupture of some cardiovascular structure. In the absence of a history of trauma, the most probable candidates for rupture or dissection are the aorta and the sinuses of Valsalva. In most cases of dissection of the aorta, there is a history of some connective tissue disorder such as Marfan syndrome, and dissection, even in those affected, is almost unknown before puberty. Dissection of the aorta can occasionally be diagnosed by transthoracic ultrasound, but often other diagnostic methods are required, such as transesophageal echocardiography or angiography. Rupture of the sinuses of Valsalva is also a rare condition that occurs sporadically, but it is usually easily diagnosed on two-dimensional examination by identifying the abnormal flow coming from the sinus. This is more common in older individuals and is, therefore, discussed in more detail in Chapter 6.

Fatigue

Fatigue is a common complaint among children (and their parents!) but is seldom cardiac in cause. There is much confusion about fatigue as a symptom; the term can mean many different and distinct symptoms. Cardiac fatigue is usually manifested as decreased exercise tolerance or shortness of breath with exercise. Notably, children seldom complain of shortness of breath but complain of fatigue instead. So if we substitute "fatigue or shortness of breath during exercise" for "fatigue," we can more easily identify the physiological causes of fatigue. Chronic fatigue, waking up tired, tiredness at the end of the day, depression, and even boredom may all be referred to as fatigue but do not have a cardiac cause. For fatigue to have a cardiac cause, there should be abnormal cardiac function. This can be due to any of a number of causes, including ventricular dysfunction, shunts, or valvular disease (Box 5–9).

Any type of ventricular dysfunction can present as fatigue. This includes any form of cardiomyopathy, from either systolic dysfunction, such as with dilated cardiomyopathies (Fig. 5–14; see also color figure), or diastolic dysfunction, as with hypertrophic cardiomyopathy. In either case, there will be a reduced cardiac reserve or reduced capacity for the heart to increase the cardiac output to match demand. Because the limiting factor in exercise tolerance in normal individuals is the maximum cardiac output, reduction will lead to a diminished exercise capacity. There will also be an increase in the diastolic filling pressure, leading to increased pulmonary venous pressure. This causes shortness of breath.

An extremely uncommon cause of left ventricular dysfunction in children is silent ischemic disease. Potential causes of ischemia are outlined under Chest Pain.

It is also possible to have a decrease in cardiac reserve, although the actual cardiac output is high or normal. This can occur if there is an increase in the baseline demand on the heart because of shunts or valvular disease. The types of shunt are the same as for an acyanotic defect (i.e., atrial septal defect, ventricular septal defect, and patent ductus arteriosus). Any type of valvular insufficiency will increase the volume load on the heart, increasing the stroke volume, but without an increase in cardiac output. Because the heart has to work harder to achieve a normal output, its ability to increase output will be limited.

Occasionally, a child may be clinically acyanotic but have a cyanotic type of defect. In this case, the presenting symptom may be fatigue. There are two potential causes for this lack of cyanosis. The first is the degree of right-to-left shunting, which may be variable depending on the individual physiology. For example, if a child has tetralogy of Fallot but has only moderate-to-severe stenosis of the pulmonary outflow, there may be a predominant left-to-right shunt across the ventricular septal defect and little or no cyanosis (Fig 5–15; see also color figure).

The second cause for a lack of cyanosis with a cyanotic defect is that absolute amount of desaturated hemoglobin is not sufficient to create the clinical appearance of cyanosis (Fig. 5–16), even though the oxygen saturation is low owing to anemia.

Stenotic valvular disease can also limit cardiac reserve. The pressure gradient across a stenotic valve is a function of the square of the flow across the valve, so that with a doubling in cardiac output, the gradient will increase fourfold. This can rapidly limit the maximum cardiac output that can be obtained.

How Can They Be Ruled Out (or In)?

The examination to rule out cardiac causes of fatigue is the same screening examination as mentioned previously but with

---

BOX 5–9
POTENTIAL CARDIAC CAUSES OF EXERTION-INDUCED FATIGUE

Dilated cardiomyopathy

Hypertrophic cardiomyopathy

Shunts

Aortic stenosis

Pulmonic stenosis

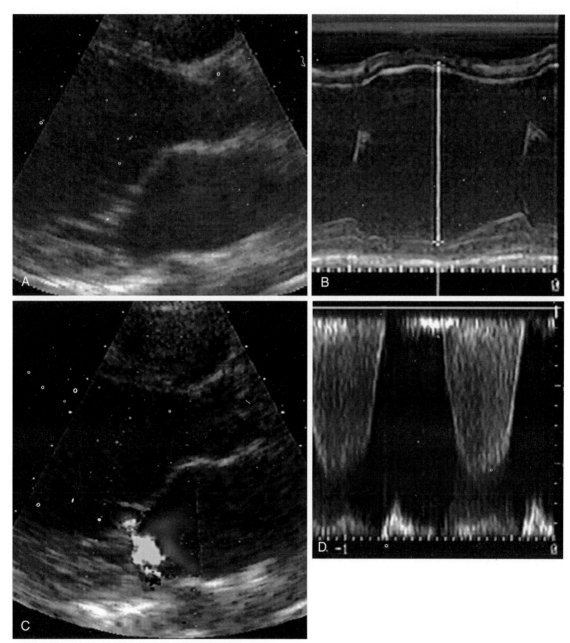

Figure 5–14. Images from an 8-year-old girl who presented with decreased exercise tolerance. A, The parasternal long-axis view, with marked left ventricular dilatation. B, An M-mode tracing, with the cursors marking the left ventricular end-diastolic dimension, which was 61 mm. This is markedly over the upper limit of normal for adults. The next recordings show mitral regurgitation by color Doppler (C; see also color figure) and continuous-wave Doppler (D). The combination of modest color flow and modest density on the continuous wave leads to a grading of mild to moderate mitral regurgitation.

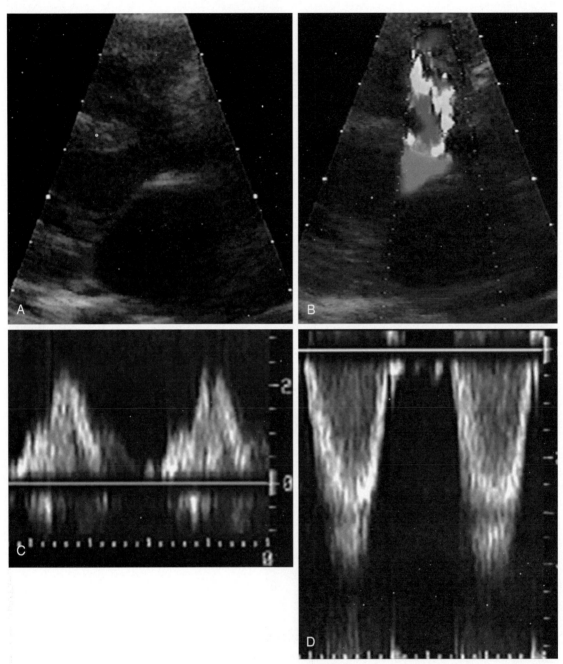

Figure 5–15. Images from a 1-year-old toddler with tetralogy of Fallot. *A,* A parasternal long-axis view demonstrating the malalignment ventricular septal defect, with the aorta overriding the ventricular septum. *B,* The flow across the defect from left to right, which is low velocity because the defect is not restrictive. *C,* The quantitative low velocity of flow across the defect, using high-pulse-repetition-frequency (HPRF) Doppler. *D,* The peak velocity through the pulmonic valve, also using HPRF Doppler, demonstrating a peak velocity of about 4.5 m/s, corresponding to a peak gradient of 80 mm Hg.

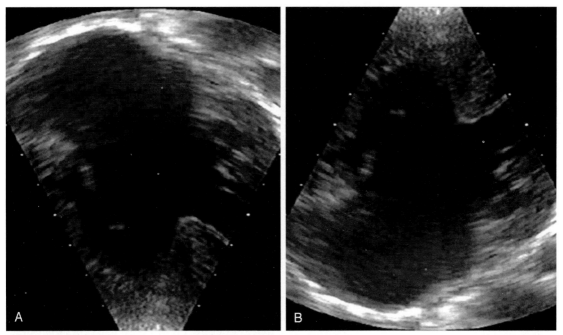

Figure 5–16. Images from a 7-year-old with fatigue. The images are identical but presented in different orientations. A, The pediatric orientation. B (see also color figure), The adult orientation. Both are apical four-chamber views. A large defect encompasses the atrial septum, the ventricular septum, and the straddling atrioventricular valve. This is a large atrioventricular septal defect.

some minor modifications of what we are looking for (Box 5–10).

Normal chamber size and thickness: any shunt or valvular regurgitation sufficient to cause fatigue should cause an increase in chamber size. Similarly, any significant systolic dysfunction should be accompanied by ventricular dilation, and hypertrophy should be easily detected on the two-dimensional examination.

Normal ventricular wall function: resting ischemia or infarction may cause wall function abnormalities. These are best detected by defects in wall thickening rather than "wall motion," because lateral motion of the heart can cause confusion in the interpretation of wall motion.

No evidence of increased velocities in the aortic or pulmonic outflows: this would rule out significant stenosis of these valves.

Normal right ventricular systolic pressure: this rules out pulmonary hypertension or peripheral pulmonic stenosis.

No evidence for ventricular septal defects: these should be looked for, but unless there is evidence for ventricular dilation or pulmonary hypertension, it is unlikely that this could be the cause of fatigue.

No evidence for a patent ductus arteriosus: the argument for this is similar to that for ventricular septal defects.

No evidence for atrial septal defects: the argument is similar to that for ventricular septal defects and patent ductus arteriosus.

No evidence for an aortic coarctation: this must be checked from the suprasternal notch.

No evidence for significant valvular regurgitation: this is assessed by two-dimensional imaging, HPRF or CW Doppler, and color Doppler (see Chapter 6, Left Heart). Again, regurgitation of the tricuspid, pulmonic, and mitral valves can be present in trace to mild quantities in normal individuals. Aortic regurgitation is always an abnormal finding. Tricuspid and mitral insufficiency may cause systolic murmurs, and pulmonic and aortic regurgitation can cause diastolic murmurs.

BOX 5–10

SUFFICIENT EXAMINATION TO RULE OUT A CARDIAC SOURCE OF FATIGUE OR CHEST PAIN

Ventricles

  Normal in size

  Normal function

  Normal wall thickness

Atria

  Normal size

  No evidence for atrial septal defect

Atrioventricular valves

  No significant insufficiency

  No stenosis

Semilunar valves

  No significant insufficiency

  No stenosis

Great vessels

  No coarctation

  No evidence for sinus of Valsalva aneurysm

Other

  No pericardial thickening or effusion

  No elevation of right ventricular peak
  systolic pressure

HYPERTENSION

Fortunately, hypertension is rare in children. It is almost always associated with another, serious disease such as renal failure. The cardiovascular congenital cause of hypertension is coarctation of the aorta, which is sometimes first detected when the child is noted to have hypertension.

Consequences of Hypertension on the Heart

The consequences of hypertension for the heart in children are very similar to those in adults. Ventricular hypertrophy is a prominent feature; secondary ventricular relaxation abnormalities result in a diastolic filling abnormality.

EFFECTS ON THE HEART OF OTHER DISEASE

Several other conditions are not considered to be primarily cardiac but may have significant cardiac consequences. In such cases, an echocardiographic examination may be extremely helpful in assessing whether cardiac involvement has occurred and whether therapy, or a change in therapy, is necessary.

Muscular Dystrophy

Duchenne's muscular dystrophy almost always affects ventricular function, causing a dilated cardiomyopathy. In fact, left ventricular failure is frequently the cause of death in children affected with this disorder.

Evaluation is the same as for other forms of ventricular dysfunction, with examination of the chamber size and function; the latter is assessed by either fractional shortening or ejection fraction.

Viral Disease With Myocardial Involvement

The question of viral myocarditis may arise in a child who has a viral illness and who experiences cardiac rhythm disturbances. Echocardiographically, there are primarily two possible presentations of viral myocarditis. The first, and most common, is a global systolic dysfunction, with ventricular dilation and reduction in systolic function. The degree of dysfunction can vary markedly with the course of the illness; some patients have an acute reduction in ventricular function and gradual improvement after that, and others have continuous gradual deterioration. It is extremely difficult to predict the ultimate degree of ventricular impairment during the acute phase of the disease. The other, much less common, form is segmental wall function abnormalities, which may be more reminiscent of ischemic disease. The significance of these differences is uncertain.

In either of these forms, the global ventricular function is perhaps the most important parameter to follow. Secondary problems that may occur and complicate the situation are intraventricular clots, valvular regurgitation, and pulmonary hypertension, all of which may be assessed echocardiographically. The beneficial effects of treatment may also be evaluated echocardiographically, by observing reduction in chamber size, regurgitant degree, and pulmonary hypertension.

Cystic Fibrosis and Other Lung Disease

Cystic fibrosis is a progressive lung disease affecting children and young adults. There is no associated congenital heart defect, but there is often pulmonary hypertension resulting from the lung disease. On echocardiographic examination, the main points to look for are the right-sided systolic pressure as assessed by tricuspid regurgitation, pulmonary diastolic pressure as assessed by pulmonic insufficiency, and right ventricular hypertrophy. Other points that may be of importance are whether there is a right-to-left shunt across a patent foramen ovale.

Cancer Chemotherapy

Certain forms of cancer chemotherapy can be damaging to the heart. Although they are very effective against some malignancies, the most damaging are a class of chemotherapy agents called the anthracyclines, which include doxorubicin (Adriamycin) and daunorubicin (Cerubidine). The cardiac damage is in the form of ventricular dysfunction, which is progressive with higher doses of the medication. At low doses, the effect is not detectable. Once there is detectable damage, however, the effect of any additional doses could be catastrophic.

For this reason, many centers perform regular checks of cardiac function before each dose of chemotherapy, so that if there is any abnormality, the subsequent dose can be reduced or eliminated altogether. To perform such a check, the primary focus is left ventricular function, which is usually assessed by measuring left ventricular dimensions and either fractional shortening or ejection fraction. It is very helpful to have baseline values for each individual, because the range of normal values is large.

Other methods may be used in the future to assess damage from chemotherapy, such as stress echocardiography or assessment of diastolic function.

Chapter 6

The Teenager, the Adult, and the Previously Diagnosed Patient

The case of the adult or the teenager with congenital heart disease can be divided into two very different clinical situations. The first, and perhaps easiest, involves the patient *without* diagnosed congenital heart disease but with symptoms or signs that suggest that a defect might be present. This situation is most similar to that addressed in the preceding chapters for other age groups. The second situation involves the patient *with* diagnosed congenital heart disease, who perhaps underwent surgery, who returns for follow-up and evaluation. This is a very diverse and complicated group of patients. Although many cases are so complex that they should probably be dealt with at centers with specialized expertise, some issues and conditions can be addressed by a wide range of diagnostic laboratories.

METHOD OF EXAMINATION

The general preparations for the echocardiographic examination of the teenager and the adult with suspected or diagnosed congenital heart disease are similar to those for any other adult patient. The main difference for teenagers is that the examiner should have a heightened sensitivity to issues of modesty and body image at this age, because these may be major issues to them. This means that special attention should be paid to covering the body as much as possible, allowing privacy when dressing and undressing, limiting access via curtains and doors, and reducing the number of people in the room. Also, even more than usual, comments about the examination that could be construed as negative (e.g., "The left ventricle doesn't look good") should be avoided.

The actual examination is similar in general to the routine adult examination, but with additional attention to detail and some additional views as needed and described next.

The screening examination and criteria are likewise similar to those for the child (Box 6–1 and Fig. 6–1). Note that this screening examination applies mainly to the patient without previously diagnosed congenital heart disease; the examination for diagnosed disease is dealt with later in this chapter.

SYMPTOMS/FINDINGS

The range of symptoms or signs that suggest otherwise undiagnosed congenital heart disease in the adult is relatively limited and very similar to that of the child. In most cases, however, the range of diagnostic possibilities is narrower because so many of the potential disorders will already have been diagnosed.

An important point that bears repeating is that when a congenital defect is found, it is important to search diligently for others because the chance of additional defects is increased significantly. In particular, there are common associations of particular defects, as outlined under Syndromes in Chapter 2. If a particular defect is identified, the potentially associated defects should be sought explicitly.

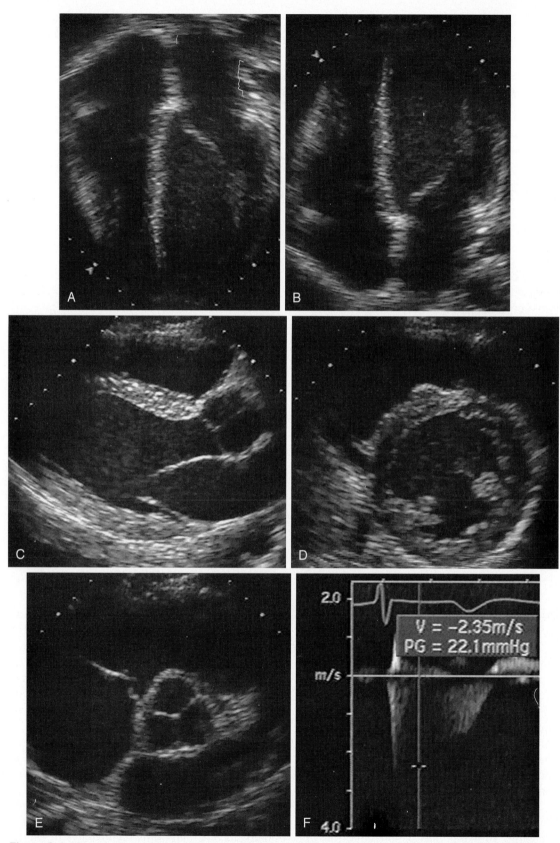

Figure 6–1. Normal echocardiogram. The four-chamber view shows normal chamber sizes (*A*, pediatric orientation; *B*, adult orientation). Normal chamber sizes are also shown in the parasternal long-axis view *(C)* and short-axis view *(D)*. A normal trileaflet aortic valve is shown in the parasternal short-axis view *(E)*, and finally normal right-sided pressures are indicated by a low-velocity tricuspid insufficiency jet *(F)*.

BOX 6–1
SURVEY EXAMINATION IN THE TEENAGER AND ADULT

Two ventricles
  Interventricular septum intact
  Left ventricle <56 mm in diameter in the adult
  Right ventricle slightly smaller than left
Two atria
  Roughly equal in size
  Left atrium <40 mm in diameter
Atrioventricular valves
  Each into respective ventricle
  Normal opening and flow
  Tricuspid displaced slightly toward apex
  Mild tricuspid insufficiency common
Semilunar valves
  Each from respective ventricle
  Normal opening and flow
  Pulmonic valve anterior
  Mild pulmonic insufficiency normal
Great arteries
  Pulmonary artery and aorta cross
  No evidence for ductal flow
  No flow acceleration in aorta or pulmonary arteries
Other
  Right ventricular pressure estimate <28 mm Hg

and aortic coarctation (Box 6–2). All of these are readily diagnosed on the screening examination.

As we expect on the basis of the physiology, we see an enlargement of the right side of the heart with an atrial septal defect. This is a very valuable tip-off, because direct imaging of the atrial septum may be difficult in the adult, and there are several potential false-positive diagnoses for atrial septal defects. A defect in the atrial septum can be easily produced based on the beam direction. If the beam is almost parallel to the atrial septum, there will be a dropout of the signal, which can look like a defect. This is most prominent in the apical view and the parasternal view, depending on the orientation of the atrial septum. For this reason, the subcostal view is preferred for imaging the atrial septum, if images are available from this window.

The most important cause of false-positive flow that appears to cross the atrial septum is flow originating in the venae cavae. Flow from the superior vena cava may appear to cross the septum when viewed from the subcostal view. Flow from the inferior vena cava is directed toward the atrial septum by the eustachian valve and seems to "rebound" off of the septum on some views (see Fig. 5–7). If the incoming flow from the inferior vena cava is not visualized directly, it can appear to be flow across the interatrial septum, especially from the parasternal and apical views. In some cases, the eustachian valve itself can give the appearance of a septum, suggesting that there is an atrial septal defect (Fig. 6–2)

Asymptomatic Murmur

The range of possible diagnoses causing an asymptomatic systolic murmur in the young adult is similar to that of the child. The major difference is that the prevalence of functional murmurs is lower; therefore, the chance that there is true disease is increased.

The screening examination for the asymptomatic young adult with a murmur is fairly standard. The most likely pathological diagnoses include atrial septal defect, ventricular septal defect, aortic stenosis (including bicuspid aortic valve), pulmonic stenosis,

BOX 6–2
MOST COMMON CAUSES OF ASYMPTOMATIC SYSTOLIC MURMURS IN THE TEENAGER AND THE ADULT

Atrial septal defect
Ventricular septal defect
Aortic stenosis
Pulmonic stenosis
Aortic coarctation

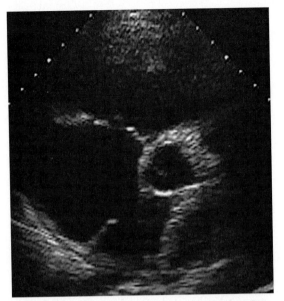

Figure 6–2. One of the sources of a "pseudo-atrialseptal defect" (ASD) is the eustachian valve, which may be prominent. In this short-axis image, the eustachian valve gives the appearance of an atrial septum. The true atrial septum is located further to the right. Doppler flow can be recorded through this "pseudo-ASD," but it will show respiratory variation opposite to a real ASD (see Fig. 6–3).

Both of these artifacts can be detected using a combination of anatomy and physiology. Identifying the flow that could be causing the false-positive diagnosis and comparing it with the flow in question will often resolve the issue by showing that it is either distinct or identical. Physiologically, the respiratory variation is opposite for the vena cava flow and atrial septal defect flow. Flow in the venae cavae increases with inspiration and decreases with expiration because of changes in the intrathoracic pressure. Flow across the interatrial septum changes in exactly the opposite manner because of the changes in right atrial pressure caused by increased or decreased filling (Fig. 6–3; see also color figure). Thus, if the flow in question decreases with inspiration and increases with expiration, it must be across an atrial septal defect, not from the venae cavae. Finally, look for the expected concomitant findings of an atrial septal defect (Box 6–3). When more of the expected findings are present, the certainty of the diagnosis becomes greater. If most of the findings are present but no shunt is visual-

ized, one should suspect partial anomalous pulmonary veins.

Although all types of ventricular septal defects may exist in patients reaching adulthood, the most likely to be first diagnosed in adulthood would probably be the perimembranous ventricular septal defect and the supracristal ventricular septal defect. Imaging of the perimembranous ventricular septal defect is best done from the parasternal window (Fig. 6–4; see also color figure), as is the imaging of the supracristal ventricular septal defect. The latter may mimic pulmonic stenosis on color Doppler examination because the disturbed flow starts just below the pulmonic valve, and turbulence continues out into the main pulmonary artery in systole. Careful pulsed-wave and continuous-wave Doppler of the direction, pattern, and timing will distinguish pulmonic stenosis from a supracristal ventricular septal defect. Perimembranous defects may close spontaneously and, in the process of closing, may develop an aneurysm in the region of the defect (Fig. 6–5).

Although muscular ventricular septal defects are common in childhood, a large proportion of these close spontaneously. When still present, they can cause an asympto-

---

BOX 6–3
POTENTIAL FINDINGS IN ATRIAL LEVEL SHUNTS (ATRIAL SEPTAL DEFECTS AND PARTIAL ANOMALOUS PULMONARY VEINS)

Ventricles
  Enlarged right ventricle
  D-shaped left ventricle
  "Paradoxical" septal motion
Atria
  Right atrial enlargement
  Flow across interatrial septum
Atrioventricular and semilunar valves
  Evidence for increased right-sided flows
Other (late appearance)
  Elevated right ventricular and pulmonary
    artery pressures

Text continued on page 145

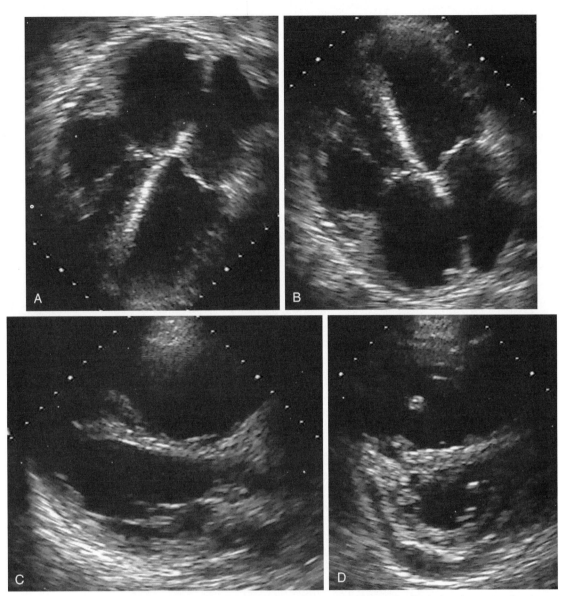

Figure 6–3. Images from a patient with an atrial secundum septal defect who had the diagnosis of primary pulmonary hypertension before this echo was performed. A, The four-chamber view in the standard pediatric orientation. B, The same view in the adult orientation. Note the right ventricular enlargement and the appearance of a defect in the atrial septum. The latter finding should be discounted because of the possibility of a false-positive image from this view. C is a long-axis view, showing the right ventricular enlargement and septal flattening. This is also shown in D in the short-axis view.

Illustration continued on following page

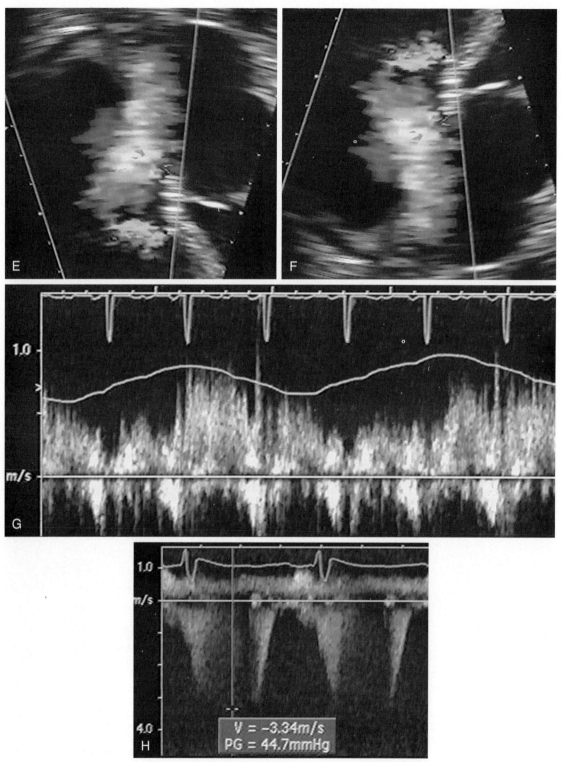

Figure 6–3 *Continued. E* (see also color figure), The flow through the atrial septal defect, from a view intermediate between an apical and subcostal view, in the pediatric orientation. *F* (see also color figure), The same image in the adult orientation. *G*, The respiratory variation of Doppler flow across the defect. The curve shows the respiratory cycle, with inspiration indicated by upward motion and expiration by downward motion. Note that the flow decreases during inspiration and increases during expiration. Finally, we assess the right-sided pressures through the tricuspid insufficiency velocity in *H*, finding that there is pulmonary hypertension with systolic pressures of at least 45 mm Hg. A calculation of the ratio of pulmonary to systemic flow on this patient yielded a value of 2.3:1.

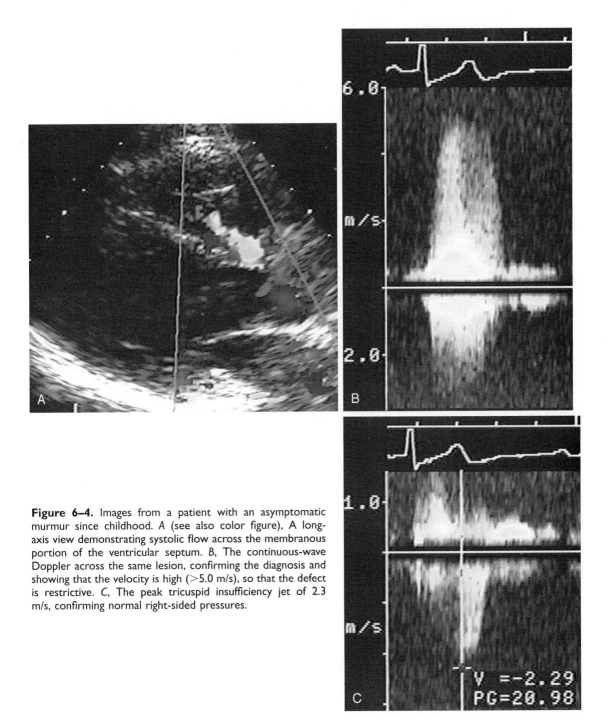

Figure 6–4. Images from a patient with an asymptomatic murmur since childhood. *A* (see also color figure), A long-axis view demonstrating systolic flow across the membranous portion of the ventricular septum. *B*, The continuous-wave Doppler across the same lesion, confirming the diagnosis and showing that the velocity is high (>5.0 m/s), so that the defect is restrictive. *C*, The peak tricuspid insufficiency jet of 2.3 m/s, confirming normal right-sided pressures.

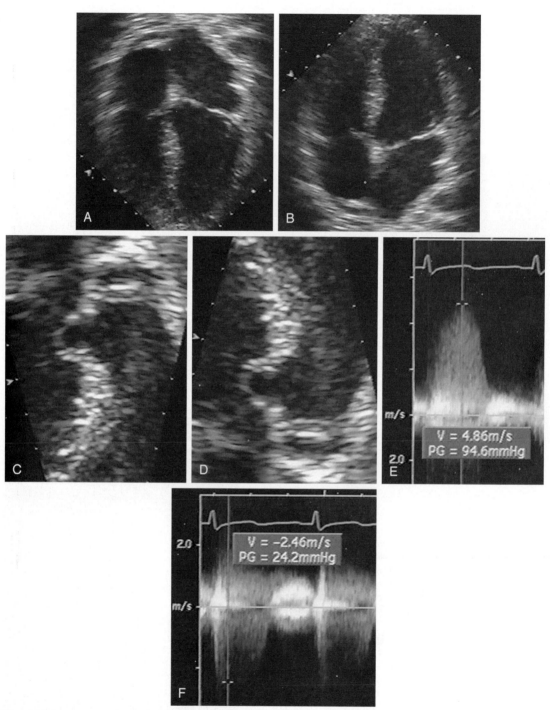

Figure 6–5. Images from another patient with a heart murmur since childhood. The four-chamber view is normal (A, pediatric orientation; B, adult orientation), but in the membranous portion of the septum from the apical long-axis view there is a defect that is almost completely closed by an aneurysm (C, pediatric orientation; D, adult orientation). The base of the defect is 1.1 cm in diameter. The remaining defect is restrictive, as demonstrated by continuous-wave Doppler of the velocity through the defect, with a peak velocity of 4.9 m/s, or 95 mm Hg (E). Low right-sided pressures are confirmed by the low velocity of the tricuspid insufficiency jet (F).

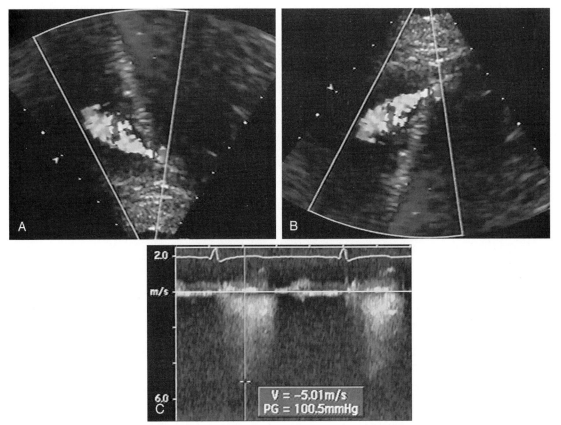

Figure 6–6. Apical four-chamber view in a patient with an asymptomatic murmur. There is clear shunting from the left ventricle to the right ventricle in the apex on the four-chamber, zoomed view (*A*, pediatric orientation [see also color figure]; *B*, adult orientation [see also color figure]). The defect is clearly restrictive, as evidenced by the continuous-wave Doppler velocity of 5.0 m/s *(C)*.

matic murmur (Fig. 6–6; see also color figure).

When a ventricular septal defect is detected, the functional significance should be determined. The key elements to evaluate are listed in Box 6–4 and are related to the volume of shunt and resulting pressure effects. Note that, in general, a *low* velocity across the defect (<4 m/s) implies either a *large* shunt or *high* pulmonary resistance or both. Aortic insufficiency is found in association with both perimembranous and supracristal ventricular septal defects up to 7% of the time. In some cases, the degree of insufficiency may be more significant than the septal defect shunt (Fig. 6–7; see also color figure).

Aortic stenosis of significant degree should be fairly easy to detect on the screening examination. Commonly, the patient will have a bicuspid aortic valve but without significant stenosis. There is usually doming of the aortic valve, and the opening of the valve is more oval than triangular (Fig. 6–8; see also color figure). There is often mild dilation of the ascending aorta, called poststenotic dilation, which can be present even when there is not a significant stenosis but there is disturbed flow through a bicuspid valve. As always, it is important to eval-

---

BOX 6–4
EVALUATION OF SEVERITY OF
VENTRICULAR SEPTAL DEFECTS

Velocity of flow across ventricular septum

Right ventricular and pulmonary artery
  pressures

Left ventricular size

Left atrial size

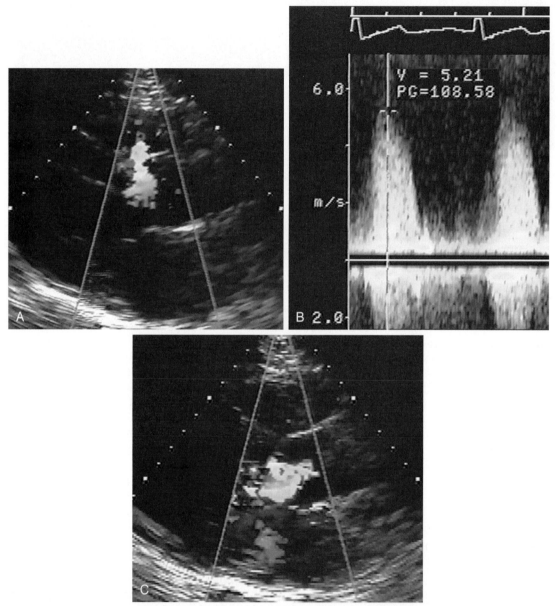

Figure 6–7. Images from a patient with a harsh systolic murmur. There is clearly a perimembranous ventricular septal defect (*A* [see also color figure]), which is restrictive, with a velocity through the defect of 5.2 m/s, for a gradient of almost 110 mm Hg *(B)*. There is also aortic insufficiency (*C* [see also color figure] and *D*), which is moderate in degree, as evidenced by late diastolic reverse flow in the descending aorta *(E)*. Normally, there is reversal of flow in the descending aorta early in diastole but not at the end.

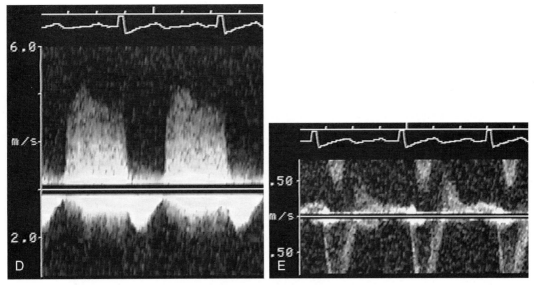

Figure 6–7 *Continued*

uate the physiology both for degree of stenosis and insufficiency (Fig. 6–9). Because there is a strong association, coarctation should also be sought.

Pulmonic stenosis of mild degree is a common cause of an asymptomatic murmur. In addition to evaluating the hemodynamic consequences, it is also important to check for possible atrial septal defect, which could be causing increased velocity of flow across a valve of normal area. Similarly to aortic stenosis, poststenotic dilation of the main pulmonary artery can occur.

Coarctation of the aorta may present with an asymptomatic murmur, although we usually associate it more with high blood pressure or pulse deficits. The most common site for an aortic coarctation, the descending aorta just distal to the left subclavian artery, is usually visible on the screening examination (Fig. 6–10; see also color figure). In assessing the severity of aortic coarctation, it is important to include the proximal velocity in the Bernoulli equation because this may be significant and if omitted would lead to a significant overestimation of the gradient.

To rule out congenital heart disease as the cause of an asymptomatic murmur, it is sufficient to identify normal ventricular size and function, normal atrial size, normal valvular function, and normal flows in the great arteries (Box 6–5). If possible, estima-

tion of the right ventricular peak systolic pressure can add reliability to the diagnosis, because elevation of the right-sided pressure not only can indicate pathology but can

---

BOX 6–5
SUFFICIENT EXAMINATION FOR ASYMPTOMATIC MURMUR

Two ventricles
  Interventricular septum intact
  Right ventricle slightly smaller than left
Two atria
  Roughly equal in size
  Left atrium <40 mm in diameter
Atrioventricular valves
  Normal opening and flow
  Mild tricuspid insufficiency common
Semilunar valves
  Normal opening and flow
  Mild pulmonic insufficiency normal
Great arteries
  No evidence for ductal flow
  No flow acceleration in aorta or
    pulmonary arteries
Other
  Right ventricular pressure estimate
    <28 mm Hg

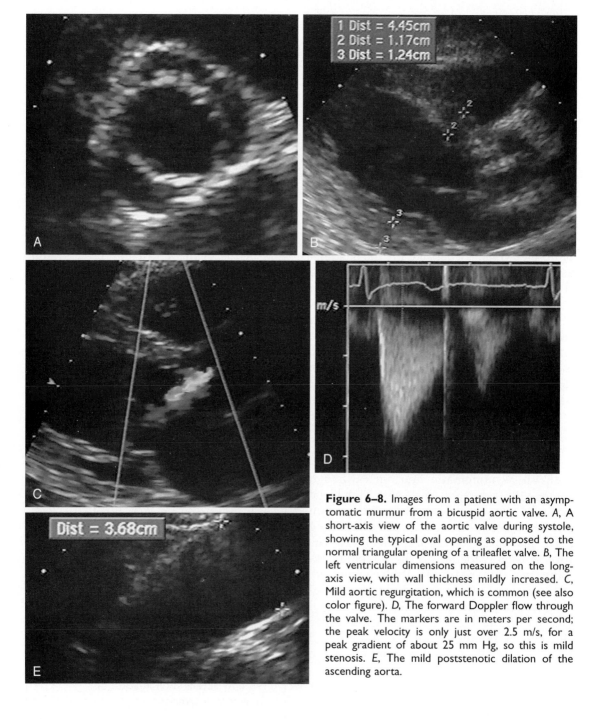

Figure 6–8. Images from a patient with an asymptomatic murmur from a bicuspid aortic valve. A, A short-axis view of the aortic valve during systole, showing the typical oval opening as opposed to the normal triangular opening of a trileaflet valve. B, The left ventricular dimensions measured on the long-axis view, with wall thickness mildly increased. C, Mild aortic regurgitation, which is common (see also color figure). D, The forward Doppler flow through the valve. The markers are in meters per second; the peak velocity is only just over 2.5 m/s, for a peak gradient of about 25 mm Hg, so this is mild stenosis. E, The mild poststenotic dilation of the ascending aorta.

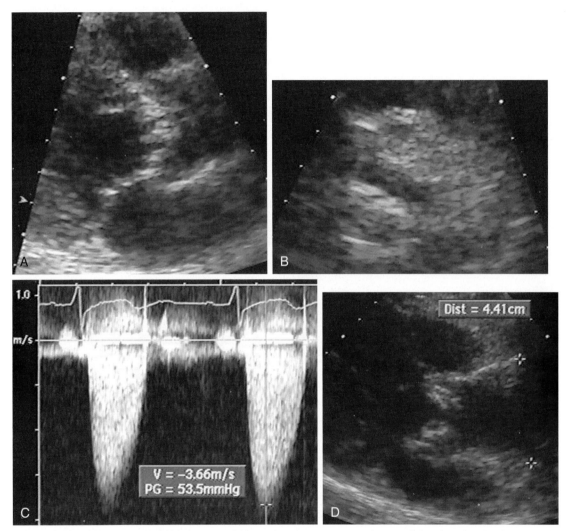

Figure 6–9. Images from another patient with an asymptomatic murmur but much harsher than in the patient in Figure 6–8. *A*, The long-axis view of the aortic valve. It is possible to see that the valve is heavily sclerotic. *B*, A short-axis view of the same valve, which is difficult to interpret because of the heavy sclerosis. The oval opening is just visible in the center of the picture, indicating that this is a bicuspid aortic valve. *C*, The transaortic continuous-wave Doppler, with a peak velocity of 3.7 m/s, for a peak gradient of 55 mm Hg. *D*, The ascending aorta with poststenotic dilation.

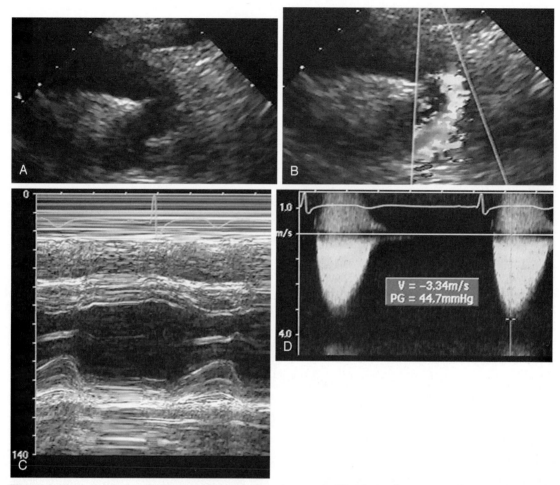

Figure 6–10. Images from a patient with hypertension and a murmur. The descending aortic arch appears somewhat tortuous (A), and there is acceleration of flow in the abnormal region (B) (see also color figure). The proximal velocity does not account for a significant portion of the gradient (C), and there is mild left ventricular hypertrophy on M-mode exam (D). This is a coarctation of the aorta with a mild to moderate gradient.

also obscure pathology, such as ventricular septal defects.

Decreased Exercise Tolerance or Enlarged Heart

Some patients present with symptoms of fatigue or cardiac enlargement on other studies such as chest x-ray film or computed tomographic examination. As noted in Chapter 5, the symptom of fatigue is subject to a wide range of interpretations. For the symptom to be related to cardiac dysfunction, there should be decreased exercise tolerance with or without dyspnea. General-

ized fatigue, not related to exertion, rarely is a sign of cardiac disease.

The range of congenital defects that will cause cardiac enlargement or exercise intolerance in the teenager or the adult without being diagnosed earlier is somewhat limited. In all cases, there will be an abnormality on the screening echocardiographic examination. The potential causes are conveniently divided according to the location of the abnormalities found on the screening examination (Box 6–6).

Left Side of Heart

The left ventricle may be enlarged, or hypertrophic, or there may be evidence for obstruction. An enlarged left ventricle can be due to volume overload or decreased left ventricular function, whereas hypertrophy may be primary or secondary to pressure overload. Obstructions may occur to left ventricular inflow and outflow.

Volume overload in this age group is usually caused by either aortic or mitral insufficiency. In either case, the findings are that the left ventricle is enlarged. However, early in the course, it will have normal or hyperdynamic function; and late in the course, there can be decreased systolic function of the left ventricle. In either case, the valvular insufficiency will be easy to see on Doppler examination. Isolated congenital aortic insufficiency is usually due to a bicuspid aortic valve, whereas isolated congenital mitral insufficiency is most probably due to a

cleft mitral valve, which is the minimal type of an endocardial cushion defect.

A caveat that should be repeated here is not to judge the severity of the insufficiency solely by the appearance on color Doppler. There are many factors that influence the appearance on color Doppler independent of the true severity. These can cause either overestimation of the severity or, more rarely, underestimation. A good rule of thumb is to look for signs of physiological compromise before identifying insufficiency as moderate or greater. For aortic insufficiency, these signs are left ventricular dilation, end-diastolic flow reversal in the descending aorta, and rapid deceleration of the aortic insufficiency velocity (Fig. 6–11). For mitral insufficiency, these signs are left ventricular dilation, left atrial dilation, and blunting or reversal of the systolic flow in the pulmonary veins (Fig. 6–12).

A dilated left ventricle with reduced systolic function may be secondary to long-standing valvular insufficiency. More commonly, however, it is due to systolic dysfunction, either a primary cardiomyopathy or a secondary cardiomyopathy (Fig. 6–13; see also color figure). The appearance on echocardiography is very similar for these two groups, and additional clinical information is necessary to differentiate them. Congenital disorders causing cardiomyopathy, such as muscular dystrophy, also give a similar echocardiographic appearance.

Another rare cause of left ventricular dysfunction, resulting in an enlarged heart, is an anomalous coronary artery or coronary fistula. If one of the coronary arteries originates from the pulmonary artery, there is retrograde flow in that artery and relative ischemia of the region supplied by that artery. This can result in chest pain or decreased function and symptoms of heart failure. This can also occur if there is a large fistula to a low-pressure chamber. It can be difficult to identify this abnormality, but on some occasions the anomalous vessel can be identified emptying into the pulmonary artery or elsewhere. In rare instances, the collateral vessels connecting the normal to the aberrant coronary are so large that they themselves can be visualized (Fig. 6–14).

BOX 6–6
CLASSIFICATION OF POTENTIAL FINDINGS IN ENLARGED HEART/ DECREASED EXERCISE TOLERANCE

Left side of heart
  Enlarged left ventricle
    Aortic insufficiency
    Mitral insufficiency
    Decreased systolic function
    Anomalous coronary arteries
  Hypertrophic left ventricle
    Aortic stenosis
    Coarctation
    Asymmetric hypertrophy
Right side of heart
  Enlarged right ventricle
    Atrial septal defect
    Partial anomalous pulmonary veins
    Pulmonic insufficiency
    Tricuspid insufficiency
    Ebstein's anomaly
  Hypertrophic right ventricle
    Pulmonic stenosis
    Pulmonary hypertension

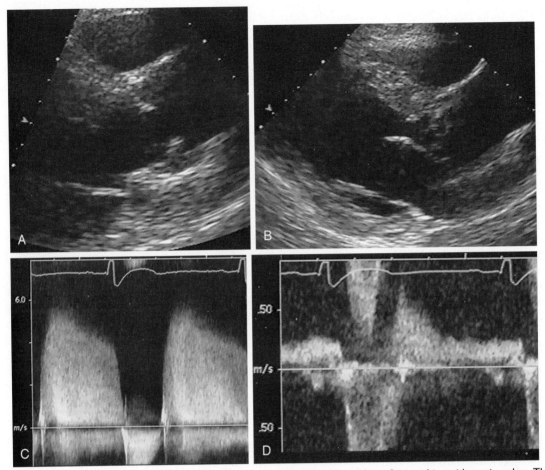

Figure 6–11. This patient has moderately severe aortic insufficiency resulting from a bicuspid aortic valve. The long-axis view of the aortic valve in systole shows the doming caused by incomplete opening *(A)*. The full long-axis view shows the mild left ventricular dilation, with a left ventricular end-diastolic dimension of 62 mm Hg *(B)*. Continuous-wave Doppler from the apex shows the aortic insufficiency, with a sharp deceleration slope *(C)*. Finally, there is end-diastolic flow reversal in the descending aortic flow measured by pulsed Doppler *(D)*.

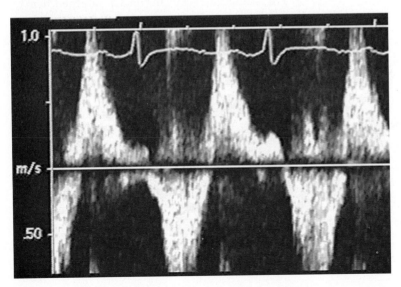

Figure 6–12. This is a Doppler tracing from the left upper pulmonary vein of a patient with severe mitral regurgitation. It is recorded during a transesophageal echocardiogram; therefore, the tracings are clearer than normally obtained on a transthoracic study. During systole, there is flow into the pulmonary vein (downward), which represents reversal caused by the increase in left atrial pressure.

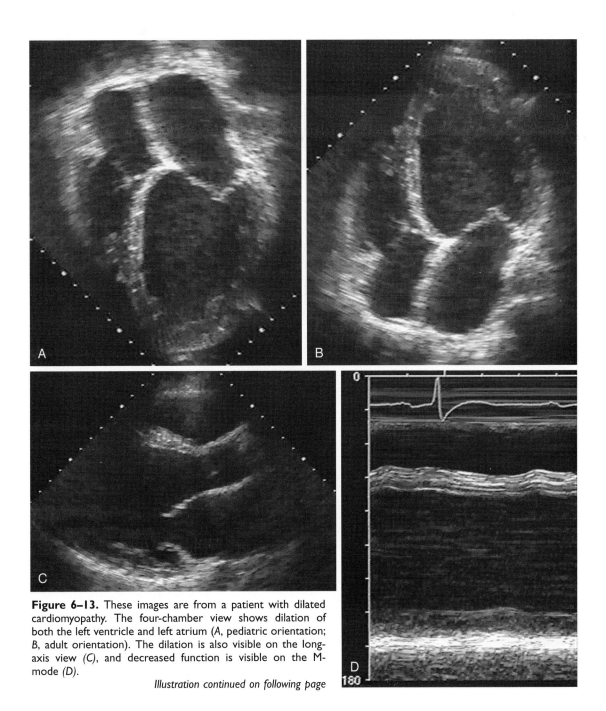

Figure 6–13. These images are from a patient with dilated cardiomyopathy. The four-chamber view shows dilation of both the left ventricle and left atrium (*A*, pediatric orientation; *B*, adult orientation). The dilation is also visible on the long-axis view (*C*), and decreased function is visible on the M-mode (*D*).

Illustration continued on following page

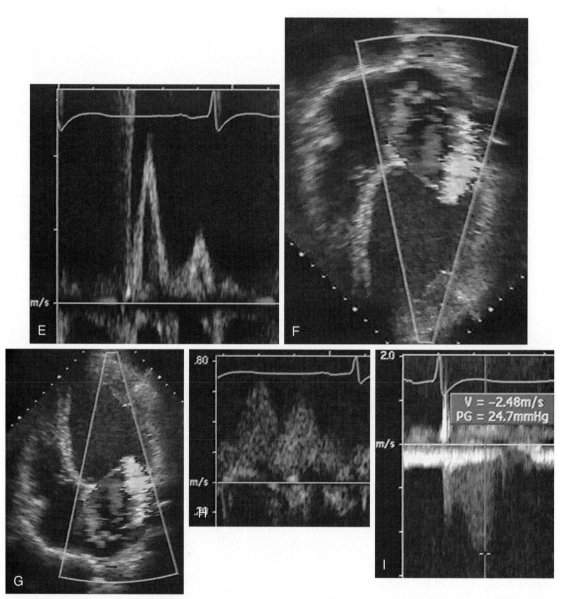

Figure 6–13 *Continued.* The transmitral Doppler shows a diminished atrial wave, indicating decreased left ventricular compliance *(E)*, and there is mitral regurgitation *(F* [see also color figure], pediatric orientation; *G* [see also color figure], adult orientation). The degree of insufficiency cannot be very great because the pulmonary venous flow is normal *(H)*; flow during systole is more prominent than during early diastole. Finally, right-sided pressures are normal, as shown by the tricuspid insufficiency velocity *(I)*.

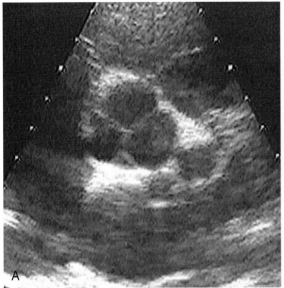

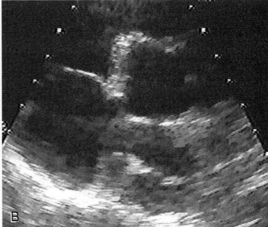

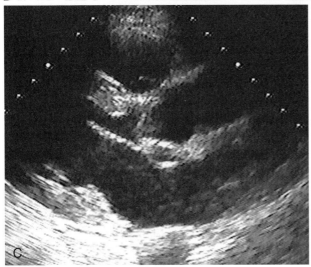

Figure 6–14. Images from a patient who originally presented with an asymptomatic continuous murmur and was found to have a left coronary artery to right atrial fistula on echocardiography. The parasternal short-axis view at the aortic level shows two echolucent areas below and to the right on the image from the aortic valve *(A)*. The upper area is actually the dilated left coronary artery, and the lower area is the fistula. The fistula dilated considerably as it coursed toward the right atrium and behind the aortic annulus. It can be seen entering the right atrium by slightly angulating the transducer from the same parasternal short-axis view *(B)*. In the long-axis view, the fistula can be seen posterior to the aortic annulus *(C)*.

Hypertrophy of the left ventricle can be primary or secondary. Whatever the cause of hypertrophy, there is impaired relaxation of the left ventricle, which can result in increased filling pressures and symptoms. Pressure overload is usually due to aortic stenosis or coarctation but may also be due to systemic hypertension. It usually causes hypertrophy long before causing dilation. Fatigue may be due to decreased reserve and maximum output, or dyspnea may result from the impaired filling because of the hypertrophy. In hypertrophic cardiomyopathy, the primary form of hypertrophy, the thickening is usually asymmetric and may cause an obstruction to outflow from the left ventricle. The relationship between this obstruction and the presence of symptoms is controversial.

Right Side of Heart

As is true for the left side of the heart, the right side can be enlarged, or hypertrophic, and there may be evidence for obstruction. The most significant difference is that isolated right ventricular dysfunction is quite rare, and when it is present it is not strictly a congenital defect.

Enlargement of the right ventricle can be due to volume overload or systolic dysfunction, as with the left ventricle. Volume overloads are caused by pulmonic insufficiency, tricuspid insufficiency, or shunts at the atrial level or before. In all of these cases, enlargement of the right ventricle is evident and in some cases enlargement of the right atrium as well. If there is no identifiable cause of right ventricular enlargement, such as valvular insufficiency or atrial septal defects, but systolic function appears normal, one should be suspicious of partial anomalous pulmonary veins.

Hypertrophy of the right ventricle is virtually always due to pressure overload. Pressure overload of the right side of the heart is readily diagnosed by echocardiography. The major causes are pulmonic stenosis, pulmonary hypertension from shunts, and pulmonary hypertension from pulmonary disease (cor pulmonale). Pressure overload may also be secondary to left-sided problems such as mitral stenosis or insufficiency. In any case, we should find evidence for increased right ventricular pressures on the basis of the velocity of the tricuspid insufficiency jet. If there is valvular pulmonic stenosis or infundibular stenosis, we should be able to detect the increased velocity of flow at the valve or the pulmonary outflow tract as well. If we are unable to detect any gradients at either of these sites, and we have evidence for increased pulmonary pressures, the diagnosis must either be pulmonary hypertension or peripheral pulmonic stenosis.

This sort of evaluation is important for patients with the diagnosis of primary pulmonary hypertension, because a congenital heart defect may be the actual cause, and it still may be correctable. The most common congenital defects that are easily missed are atrial level shunts, including secundum atrial septal defects (see Fig. 6–3), sinus venosus defects (Fig. 6–15; see also color figure), and patent ductus arteriosus (Fig. 6–16).

Right ventricular systolic dysfunction is rare in congenital heart disease outside of the conditions just identified. If it is present, one should be suspicious of right ventricular dysplasia, which is not strictly congenital, although clearly there is some type of predisposition. The primary importance of this diagnosis is the risk of serious ventricular arrhythmias.

The sufficient examination to rule out a congenital source of decreased exercise tolerance or enlarged heart is listed in Box 6–7. Although it is not a congenital problem, pericardial effusion should be sought because this can also cause the appearance of an enlarged heart on x-ray.

Hypertension

Aortic coarctation can cause systemic hypertension (see Fig. 6–10) and, therefore, should be sought in patients undergoing echocardiography as part of the evaluation of hypertension.

Chest Pain

The incidence of pathological chest pain in teenagers and young adults is low, espe-

---

BOX 6–7
SUFFICIENT EXAMINATION FOR
DECREASED EXERCISE TOLERANCE/
ENLARGED HEART

Two ventricles
  Normal left ventricular size and function
  Right ventricle slightly smaller than left
Two atria
  Roughly equal in size
  Left atrium <40 mm in diameter
Atrioventricular valves
  Normal opening and flow
  Mild tricuspid insufficiency common
Semilunar valves
  Normal opening and flow
  Mild pulmonic insufficiency normal
Great arteries
  No flow acceleration in aorta or
    pulmonary arteries
Other
  Right ventricular pressure estimate
    <28 mm Hg
  No significant pericardial effusion

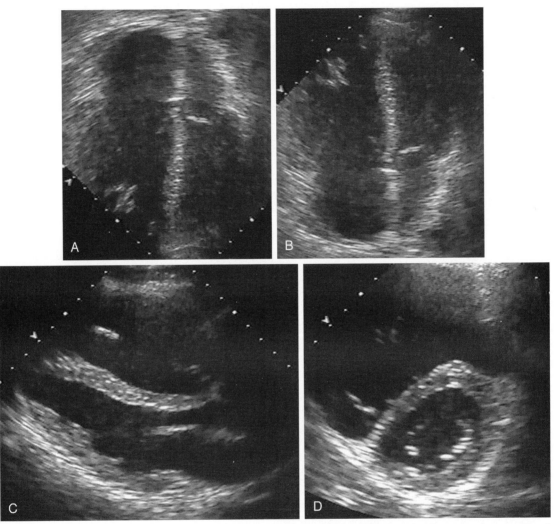

Figure 6–15. This patient had murmur and decreased exercise tolerance. The four-chamber view shows a dilated right ventricle (*A*, pediatric orientation; *B*, adult orientation). Right ventricular volume overload is evident by dilation of the right ventricle and flattening of the septum on the long-axis *(C)* and short-axis *(D)* views.

Illustration continued on following page

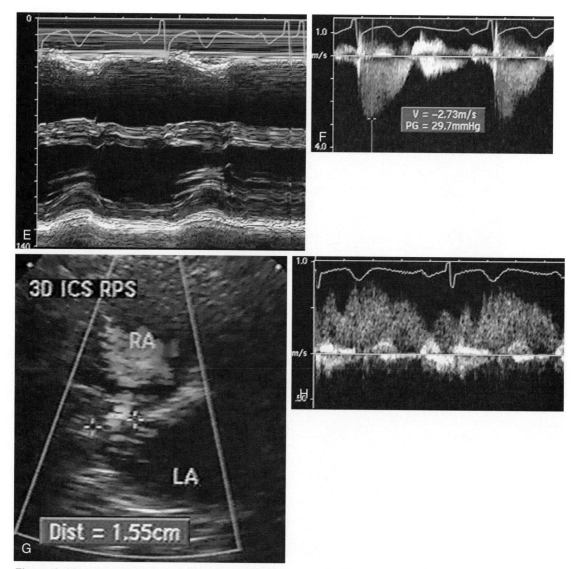

Figure 6–15 *Continued.* There is a paradoxical septal motion on the M-mode recording *(E)*. There is mild elevation of the right ventricular pressures based on the tricuspid insufficiency velocity *(F)*. From an unusual location, it was possible to demonstrate flow across a sinus venosus atrial septal defect with color flow *(G* [see also color figure]) and pulsed Doppler *(H)*. It is not always possible to demonstrate a sinus venosus defect on transthoracic studies, so in the presence of right ventricular dilation and signs of volume overload without a clear cause, a transesophageal echo may be necessary.

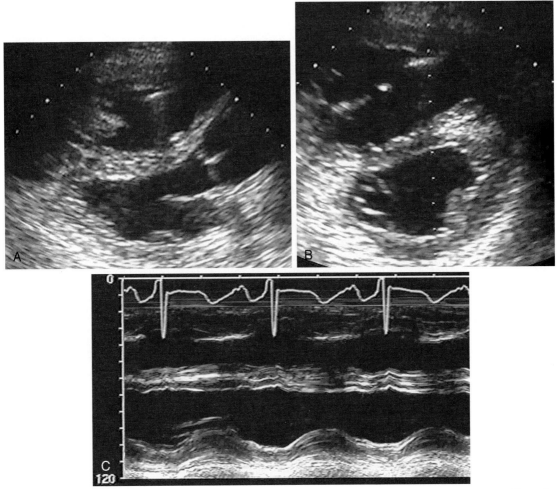

Figure 6–16. Images from a patient presenting with the diagnosis of primary pulmonary hypertension. The right ventricle is dilated and hypertrophic in both the long-axis *(A)* and short-axis *(B)* views. The interventricular septum is flattened but does not show the same paradoxical septal motion on M-mode as the sinus venosus atrial defect in Figure 6–15 *(C)*.

Illustration continued on following page

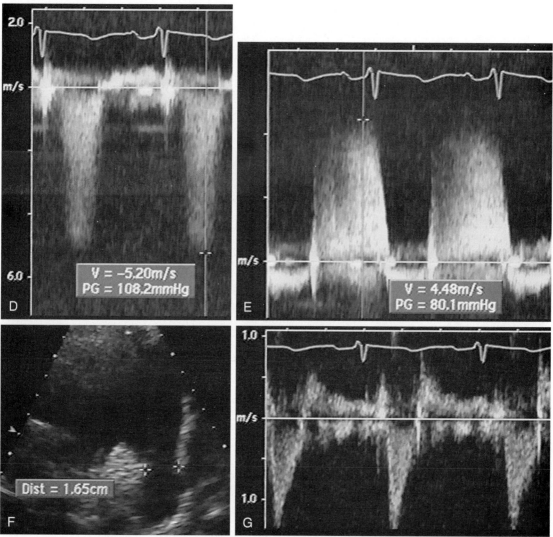

Figure 6–16 *Continued.* There is very high pulmonary pressure, as shown by the tricuspid insufficiency velocity of 5.2 m/s *(D)* and the pulmonary insufficiency velocity jet of 4.5 m/s *(E)*. A patent ductus arteriosus was found (*F*, parasternal view with main pulmonary artery superior, ductus marked with calipers, and descending aorta below), which was made more difficult to detect because there was bidirectional shunting, of low velocity, as shown by the pulsed Doppler recording in the ductus *(G)*. Unfortunately, this patient had irreversible pulmonary hypertension secondary to the ductus and could not undergo repair.

cially compared with that among older adults in whom atherosclerosis is common. In the teenager and the young adult with chest pain, ischemia is usually thought of as the prime cause on the differential diagnosis, although the etiologies of ischemia are generally different from those for older adults (Box 6–8). Because of this, especially in the younger age groups, the possibility of congenital heart disease being the pathological source of chest pain is higher than in older age groups.

Ischemia as a Source of Pain

The signs of ischemia resulting from congenital heart disease are similar to those of ischemia caused by atherosclerosis. Although ischemia usually causes chest pain, it can also cause exertional dyspnea or syncope. Congenital coronary lesions that can cause ischemia are coronary artery anomalies with either an abnormal course of the coronary arteries or abnormal origin. These are discussed in more detail later under Athletic Examination.

BOX 6–8

POTENTIAL CARDIAC CAUSES OF CHEST PAIN IN THE TEENAGER AND THE YOUNG ADULT

Ischemic

  Anomalous coronary arteries

  Aortic stenosis

  Kawasaki's syndrome

Mechanical disruption

  Sinus of Valsalva aneurysm

  Aortic aneurysm

  Pulmonary artery aneurysm

Other

  Dilated cardiomyopathy

  Hypertrophic cardiomyopathy

  Pulmonary hypertension

Chest pain that occurs with severe aortic stenosis is probably due to subendocardial ischemia, secondary to high demand and low perfusion. Kawasaki's syndrome can result in acquired coronary abnormalities, which may cause chest pain and even infarction.

Just as with atherosclerotic disease, the patient with ischemia from congenital heart disease may not have any findings on the resting echocardiogram, so this diagnosis cannot be ruled out with certainty. If there is a significant index of suspicion based on the history, a stress study should be performed.

Dissection/Aneurysm

The pain from dissection or a rupturing aneurysm is usually different in character and is often described as tearing or stabbing. The distinction between dissection and rupture is anatomic, in that a dissection separates anatomic planes and rupture disrupts the planes themselves. This means that in the aorta, dissections are longitudinal or circumferential disruptions, parallel to the wall structures; whereas rupture is in the radial direction across the wall structures. For either of these to occur, there

needs to be mechanical stress and usually some underlying structural weakness as well, although ruptures can occur with chest trauma without underlying weakness.

Dissections of the left side of the heart generally occur in the aorta or sinus of Valsalva and, in the case of congenital heart disease, are due to aneurysmal dilation of the corresponding structures. The sinuses of Valsalva can generally be visualized directly, and aneurysms are seen as enlargement of one or more of the sinuses (Fig. 6–17). If there is a rupture, the flow may often be visualized as well if it is not contained and is flowing into a cardiac chamber.

The aorta may be dilated because of either a weakness in the wall, as in Marfan syndrome, or flow disturbances such as poststenotic dilation. In either case, this can lead to dissection or rupture. Visualization of the ascending aorta is common in the transthoracic echocardiogram (Fig. 6–18; see also color figure), but reliable visualization of the transverse and descending aorta often requires transesophageal echocardiography.

Other findings also may be associated with dissection or rupture of the aorta, in-

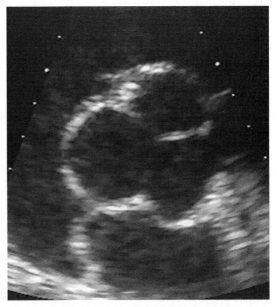

Figure 6–17. This is a short-axis view of the aortic valve in an asymptomatic patient. Note the large noncoronary sinus, which is almost 3 cm in diameter. This is an intact sinus of Valsalva aneurysm.

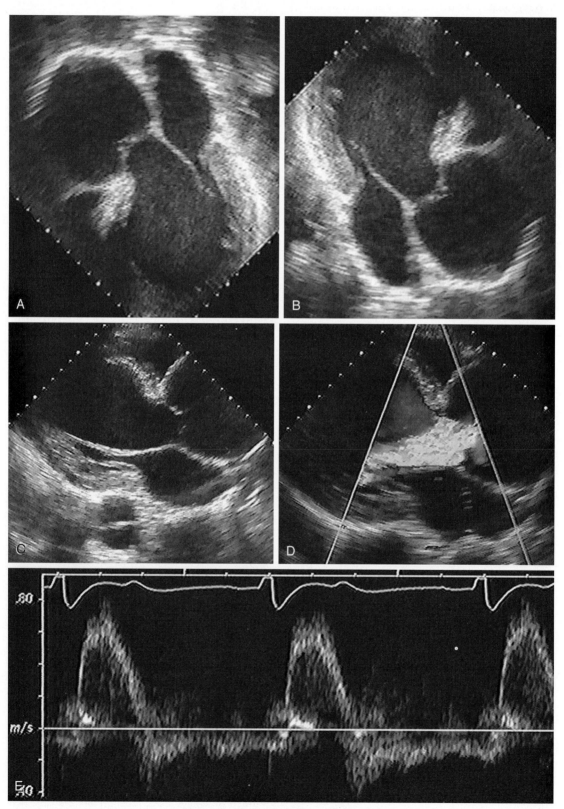

Figure 6–18. *See legend on opposite page*

cluding aortic insufficiency, pericardial effusion, and wall motion abnormalities. All of these should be sought in the patient with chest pain, although their absence does not preclude a cardiac source of pain.

The right side of the heart is more rarely the site of disease causing chest pain. This is because of the lower pressure on that side of the heart. For it to be the source of pain, there must be an elevation of pressure resulting from either pulmonic stenosis or pulmonary hypertension. Fortunately, these are easily identified on the routine examination.

One point worth mentioning is that patients who have a dilated main pulmonary artery as a result of either disease or a patch repair at surgery and who have elevated pressures in the artery as well are at higher risk for rupture. This dilation can usually be identified on the transthoracic examination and should be sought, especially in any patient with elevated right-sided pressures.

Other Diseases

Other cardiac causes of chest pain include dilated cardiomyopathy, hypertrophic cardiomyopathy, and aortic stenosis. The screening examination for the patient with chest pain is listed in Box 6–9. Note again that a resting examination is not sufficient because it cannot rule out a cardiac source of pain, and functional testing or other imaging techniques may be necessary. Although mitral valve prolapse has been cited as a "cause" of chest pain syndromes, it is my opinion that this is a spurious association. In spite of this, prolapse should be sought because the question is often raised.

BOX 6–9
(IN)SUFFICIENT EXAMINATION FOR CHEST PAIN

Two ventricles
  Normal left ventricular size and wall thickness
  Uniform left ventricular wall function
  Right ventricle slightly smaller than left
Two atria
  Roughly equal in size
  Left atrium <40 mm in diameter
Atrioventricular valves
  (No mitral valve prolapse)
Semilunar valves
  Normal opening and flow
  Mild pulmonic insufficiency normal
Great arteries
  Normal size, including sinuses of Valsalva
  No flow acceleration in aorta or pulmonary arteries
Other
  Right ventricular pressure estimate <28 mm Hg
  Proximal coronary arteries normal caliber and thickness
  Serious consideration of additional tests, such as
  stress testing for ischemia
  transesophageal imaging, magnetic resonance imaging, and computed tomography for aorta

---

ATHLETIC EXAMINATION

The examination of the patient about to participate in athletics can be divided into

---

Figure 6–18. Images from a patient with Marfan syndrome who presented with back pain and symptoms of congestive heart failure. The apical long-axis view shows the dilated left ventricle and aortic root in pediatric *(A)* and adult *(B)* orientations. The parasternal long-axis view shows left ventricular dilation and the characteristic dilation of the ascending aorta, starting at the annulus and completely involving the sinuses of Valsalva *(C)*. Note the oval echolucent area below the atrioventricular groove, which appears to be bisected horizontally. This is the descending aorta, with a dissection flap. There is aortic insufficiency *(D* [see also color figure]) which causes end-diastolic flow reversal in the abdominal aorta *(E)* and is, therefore, severe. This patient had an ascending aortic aneurysm, severe aortic insufficiency, and descending aortic dissection.

two distinct categories. One category involves the patient who has no history of heart disease but is referred for an echocardiographic examination because of either a physical finding or other suspicion of heart disease. The second involves the patient with known operated or unoperated congenital heart disease who wants to participate in sports. The considerations for these two situations are quite different, and the examination reflects this.

Patient Without Known Congenital Heart Disease

The extent of the routine preparticipation physical examination for amateur athletes, including school and organized competitive athletics as well as recreational athletics, is somewhat controversial. One of the main areas of controversy is the degree of testing for serious cardiovascular problems that is appropriate on a routine basis. Although there is no question that sudden cardiac death of a vigorous, otherwise healthy young athlete is a tragedy and that some of these individuals at risk could be identified by detailed screening examinations, the low frequency of abnormalities detected and the high cost of the screening are at the root of the controversy.

We do not need to deal with that controversy here. We will assume that the individual has been referred for an echocardiographic examination and is asymptomatic. The range of problems that may be detected is rather narrow; and although similar to the range of possible diagnoses in a patient with an asymptomatic murmur, there is a slight bias in that we are looking specifically for problems that could be hazardous during athletic activities.

Several serious conditions are frequently asymptomatic in the individual at rest or during light exercise but are more likely to cause severe symptoms or even death during exercise. These are summarized in Box 6–10. Although there are many other possible diagnoses, including those in the discussion of asymptomatic murmur, those listed are the most common diagnoses associated with significant risk. Those marked with an asterisk are associated with increased risk of death during exercise.

Significant aortic stenosis should be easy to diagnose on the basis of appearance on two-dimensional imaging and the flow velocities on Doppler. As usual, the Doppler provides an assessment of the severity, which is critical to guide further management. A related problem that can be a little more difficult to determine is a subaortic membrane. In this case, the aortic valve looks normal, but there is a high velocity on Doppler examination as a result of the membrane. In some cases, the membrane itself can be difficult to visualize; thus, the Doppler examination is critical to raising the suspicion of the diagnosis. On two-dimensional and M-mode examination of the aortic valve, there may be midsystolic closure as a result of the Venturi effect of the high velocity (Fig. 6–19; see also color figure).

Hypertrophic cardiomyopathy is a leading cardiac cause of sudden death in athletes and has both familial and isolated forms. Although this is not strictly a congenital disease, because the hypertrophy almost always develops after birth, it is included here because of its significance in the context of the sports preparticipation examination. The individuals are usually asymptomatic. This problem can be readily diagnosed by echocardiography because the hallmark is thickening of the ventricular wall. In the adult or teenager, the left ventricular wall should not exceed 11 mm in thickness. In hypertrophic cardiomyopathy,

---

BOX 6–10

ASYMPTOMATIC CONGENITAL HEART DISEASE ASSOCIATED WITH RISK DURING EXERCISE

Hypertrophic cardiomyopathy*

Anomalous coronary arteries/fistula*

Aortic aneurysm*

Sinus of Valsalva aneurysm*

Aortic stenosis*

Dilated cardiomyopathy*

Coarctation of the aorta

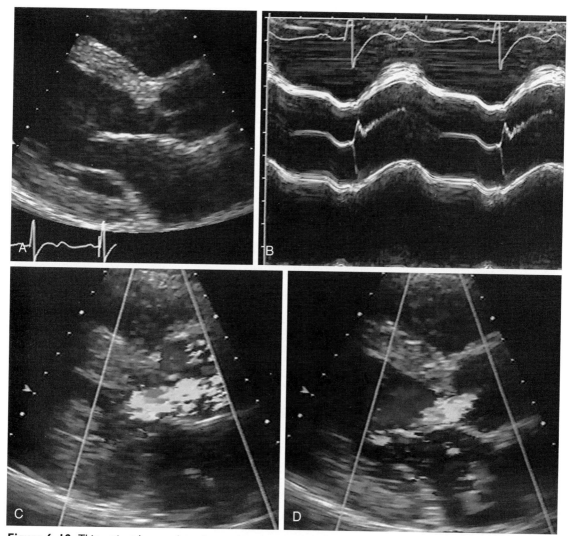

Figure 6–19. This patient has a subaortic membrane with a significant gradient. The long-axis view only hints at a subvalvular membrane *(A)*. The M-mode recording of the aortic valve shows midsystolic partial closure resulting from the Venturi effect *(B)*. Color flow mapping shows both the flow acceleration through the valve (*C* [see also color figure]) and the aortic insufficiency, which is common in this condition (*D* [see also color figure]).

Illustration continued on following page

there can be several different patterns of increased thickness. The most common is increased thickness of the interventricular septum with or without resulting left ventricular outflow obstruction. The degree of obstruction can be determined using Doppler measurement of the outflow velocity. The pattern of this type of obstruction is different from that of aortic stenosis or a subaortic membrane, because it increases during ejection, usually being greatest at end systole (Fig. 6–20). This pattern is often called a dynamic obstruction and is characteristic of a muscular obstruction. The degree of obstruction is also very dependent

on ventricular loading conditions, so that even if there is little or no obstruction at baseline, maneuvers such as Valsalva or inhaling amyl nitrate may provoke an increased gradient. I do not usually use inhalation of amyl nitrate to provoke a gradient in patients with hypertrophic cardiomyopathy because of the uncertain relationship to symptoms and prognosis, as well as the potential risk. The results of the Valsalva maneuver or even an exercise test seem more clinically relevant.

Other patients with hypertrophic cardiomyopathy may have thickening of the entire ventricular wall. Less commonly, there may

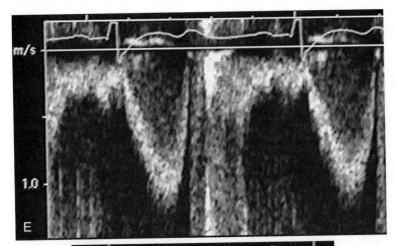

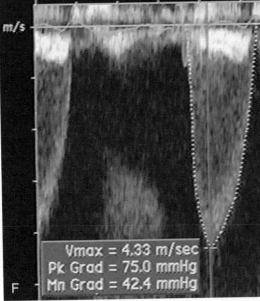

Figure 6–19 *Continued.* There is a low velocity before the area of the membrane *(E)* and a much higher velocity through the membrane *(F)*.

be focal thickening, such as only the apex (Fig. 6–21) or other walls. In any of these cases, there may be dynamic obstruction patterns of flow in the midventricle or apex.

Anomalous coronary arteries can be very difficult to diagnose, especially by resting echocardiography. Nonetheless, they are probably the second most common cardiac cause of sudden death in young athletes. There is great variability in the patterns of coronary abnormality. One type of anomaly is when one of the coronary arteries comes off the pulmonary artery instead of the aorta. The result is that there is flow out of that coronary artery into the pulmonary artery; the flow to the coronary artery from collaterals originates in the other coronary artery. This causes "a steal syndrome," in which there can be hypoperfusion of one or both coronary beds, that can worsen during exercise or other high demand. Most of these patients have symptoms of chest pain or exertional dyspnea, but they may be asymptomatic. These patients often have wall function abnormalities at rest, which become worse with exercise.

In the other type of anomaly, both coronary arteries originate from the aorta but have an abnormal course. If either of the coronary arteries passes between the aorta and the pulmonary artery, the risk of sudden death is increased. This is believed to be most risky if the left coronary artery is the one that is anomalous in this way. The

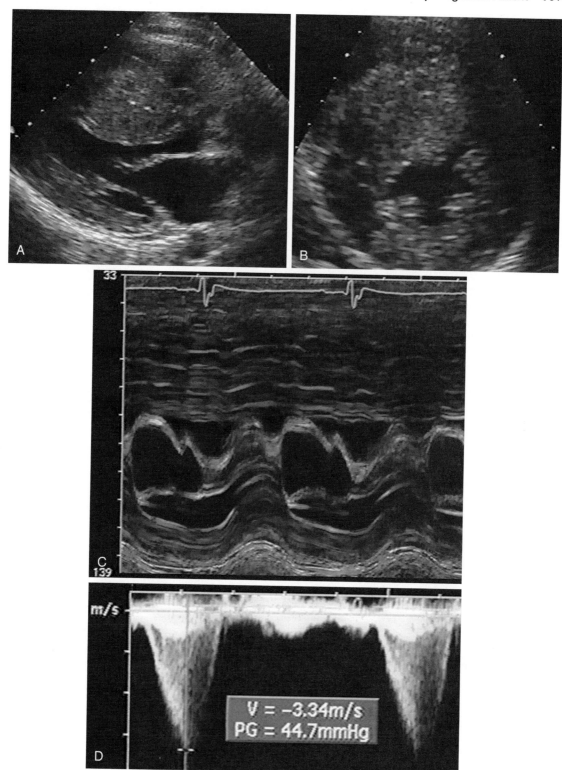

Figure 6–20. These images are from a patient with hypertrophic cardiomyopathy. There is very prominent thickening of the interventricular septum evident on the parasternal long-axis *(A)* and short-axis *(B)* views. The interventricular septum actually measured 4.4 cm. There is also systolic anterior motion of the mitral leaflets evident on M-mode *(C)*, indicating obstruction to left ventricular outflow. The continuous-wave Doppler from the apex confirms this, with a typical late-peaking flow pattern and increased velocity *(D)*. This gradient is not fixed but can vary greatly with volume status or even maneuvers such as Valsalva. This pattern of hypertrophy, predominantly involving the septum, is the most common.

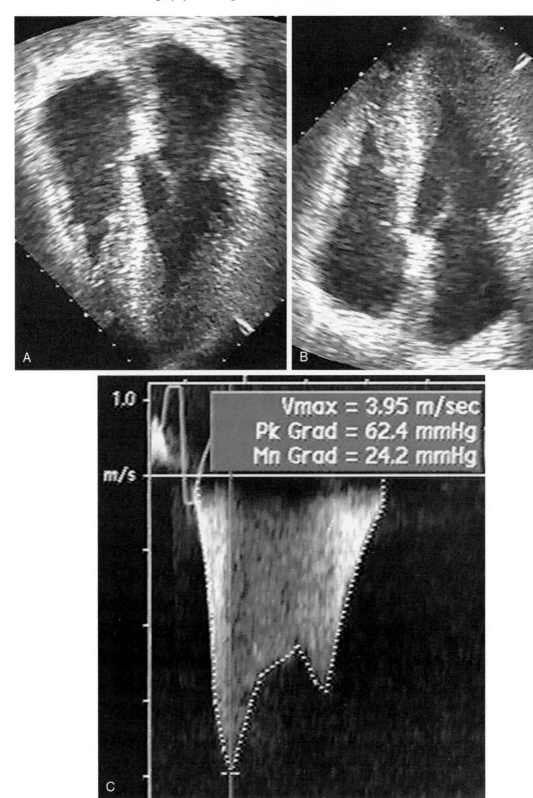

Figure 6–21. Not all patients with hypertrophic cardiomyopathy have involvement of the septum. Many patterns are possible, including hypertrophy only of the apex and apical segments, as in this patient. This is evident on these apical four-chamber views (A, pediatric orientation; B, adult orientation). There was a dynamic flow obstruction involving only the apex, shown in an apical continuous-wave recording (C).

mechanism of sudden death is believed to be compression of this anomalous artery between the pulmonary artery and aorta, resulting in ischemia. This can be very difficult to diagnose with a resting echocardiogram because the ventricular function is normal at rest. If we can identify the origins of the coronary arteries in the normal location, this makes this already very rare anomaly even less likely, but visualization of the coronary arteries cannot be performed on all patients.

The patient with a coronary fistula usually presents because of a murmur (see Fig. 6–13), but this problem can also cause a

---

BOX 6–11

(IN)SUFFICIENT PREPARTICIPATION SPORTS EXAM IN ASYMPTOMATIC PATIENT

Two ventricles

  Left ventricle <56 mm in diameter

  Uniform left ventricular wall function

  Normal wall thickness

  Right ventricle slightly smaller than left

Two atria

  Roughly equal in size

  Left atrium <40 mm in diameter

Atrioventricular valves

  Tricuspid displaced slightly toward apex

  Mild tricuspid insufficiency common

Semilunar valves

  Normal opening and flow

  Normal sinuses of Valsalva

Great arteries

  Normal size

  No flow acceleration in aorta or pulmonary arteries

Other

  (Right ventricular pressure estimate <28 mm Hg)

  Consideration of additional tests, such as

    stress testing for ischemia

    electrocardiography for long QT syndrome

---

steal syndrome similar to anomalous coronary arteries to the pulmonary trunk and can also cause ischemia.

The sinus of Valsalva aneurysm carries an increased risk of rupture, especially during high-intensity isometric exercise. The danger of such a rupture depends on where the rupture occurs. If it occurs into the right atrium, the patient will "autotransfuse" and likely be hemodynamically stable enough to be repaired. If the rupture is into the pericardium, tamponade and shock are generally rapid. Unless there is prompt surgical repair, death is likely.

Coarctation of the aorta is associated with a marked increase in the normal hypertensive response to exercise. The suprasternal view on the echocardiogram is important to view the most common location of coarctation and perform Doppler measurements.

Even if there is a completely normal, high-quality echocardiographic examination, it should be remembered that we cannot rule out all cardiac risk associated with sports participation. As noted, some of the problems, such as anomalous course of the coronary arteries, may be difficult or impossible to detect on a resting examination. In addition, patients can have potentially fatal cardiac problems that do not appear on the echocardiogram, such as long QT syndrome. So, just as for chest pain, a resting echocardiogram cannot rule out a potential problem with exercise. The findings that may be observed are listed in Box 6–11.

Examination to Determine Participation of a Patient With Congenital Heart Disease

For the patient with known congenital heart disease, whether previously operated on or not, echocardiography can be helpful to estimate the relative risk of and ability to participate in sports. This can be directly related to the degree of disorder in the physiology. The greatest increase in risk of death is related to elevations in right or left ventricular pressure, usually as a result of aortic stenosis or pulmonary vascular disease. Because the patient has known congenital heart disease, the goal of the echocardiographic examination is not to define the anatomic lesion but rather to assess the physiological impairment. This makes the screening examination somewhat different (Box 6–12). Our main concern is to assess the degree of pressure and volume stresses, where they occur, and evaluate any shunts.

The key parameters that need to be assessed are dependent on the particular diagnosis and are usually fairly easy to determine (Table 6–1). For example, if the diagnosis is a bicuspid aortic valve, the key parameters would be related to stenosis or insufficiency of the valve and would be the pressure gradient of the valve, valve area, qualitative assessment of insufficiency, left

Table 6–1. Examples of Details in Sports Examination of Patient With Congenital Heart Disease

Diagnosis	Physiology	Echo Measurements
Bicuspid aortic valve	Stenosis	Gradient, valve area, LV hypertrophy
	Insufficiency	LV size, function
Ventricular septal defect	Shunt	Gradient (restrictive), direction
		Chamber dilation or hypertrophy
		Right ventricular pressure

LV, left ventricular.

ventricular wall thickness, left ventricular dimensions, and left ventricular function.

For a ventricular septal defect, it is important to assess whether the defect is restrictive or not and the direction of shunting. If it is not restrictive, then the volume and pressure load effects on other chambers are important as well.

In situations that are unclear, it can be helpful to perform a treadmill echocardiogram both to assess the functional capacity under controlled circumstances and to assess the hemodynamic responses to exercise. A good example of this is a patient with a mild coarctation of the aorta who is normotensive at rest but who may experience an exaggerated hypertensive response with exercise.

BOX 6–12
SCREENING SPORTS EXAMINATION FOR PATIENT WITH KNOWN CONGENITAL HEART DISEASE

Ventricles
  Left ventricular size
  Left ventricular wall function
  Right and left ventricular wall thickness
  Right ventricular size
  Direction and magnitude of shunt, if present
Atria
  Atrial size
  Direction and magnitude of shunt, if present
Atrioventricular valves
  Degree of stenosis/insufficiency
Semilunar valves
  Degree of stenosis/insufficiency
Great arteries
  Direction and magnitude of ductal shunt, if present
  Degree of stenosis
Other
  Right ventricular pressure estimate
  Inferior vena cava size
  Evidence for caval obstruction

PREGNANCY AND CONGENITAL HEART DISEASE

The issue of pregnancy has two major aspects depending on whether the patient has no known congenital heart disease but has some reason to suspect a problem, usually a murmur, or whether the patient has known congenital heart disease and the risk of pregnancy must be assessed.

The cardiovascular stresses during pregnancy are many. Cardiac output increases during pregnancy, starting in the tenth week of gestation and peaking at the end of the second trimester, remaining constant after that until delivery. In addition, delivery is a strenuous activity that also involves intense Valsalva maneuvers. The Valsalva maneuver temporarily decreases venous return to the heart; therefore, venous return increases markedly immediately afterward. This can lead to right-to-left shunting for those who have diastolic left-to-right shunts and increased right-to-left shunting for those who already have a right-to-left shunt.

Murmurs Found During Pregnancy

The most common reason to suspect congenital heart disease during pregnancy is the presence of a murmur. In most cases, the murmur is due to the increased blood flow and volume during pregnancy causing increased flow through the pulmonic valve. However, another possible functional cause for a murmur during pregnancy is the mammary souffle.

Possible pathological causes of a murmur are virtually the same as for any other adult (see Box 6–2), with the added proviso that many minor defects are more easily detectable because of the high-flow state. Therefore, the sufficient examination is similar as well (see Box 6–5).

Assessing Risk of Pregnancy in Patients With Congenital Heart Disease

In patients with known congenital heart disease, one must consider many factors when assessing risk for pregnancy and delivery. These can be categorized as risks from cyanosis, shunts, and hemodynamic limitations (Table 6–2).

If a patient has cyanotic heart disease, the risks to both her and the fetus are considerable. For the fetus, there is a high incidence of fetal wastage, which increases with greater degrees of cyanosis, usually associated with a hematocrit elevation. The main risks to the mother involve paradoxical emboli, passing from the venous system to the arterial system. These can be thrombi, caused by hyperviscosity, or amniotic fluid emboli. This is true even if the individual does not have clinical cyanosis. Thus, if there is any shunt lesion, evidence for right-to-left shunting should be sought.

For noncyanotic atrial level shunts, there are similar but lower risks to the mother as a result of paradoxical emboli from straining during delivery, as noted previously. Other shunts are mainly important to the degree that they affect the hemodynamics and reserve. A major additional risk is present if there is pulmonary hypertension and especially if there is dilation of the pulmonary artery. This can lead to cardiovascular collapse, rhythm disturbances, and even pulmonary rupture during the straining associated with delivery.

Other lesions are important to the degree that they limit functional reserve, and therefore, limit the reserve available for the added demands of pregnancy and delivery. For example, a patient with significant aortic insufficiency will have already used up some of the cardiac reserve to deal with the regurgitant volume. This will limit what is available for the volume stress of pregnancy

Table 6–2. Lesions and Associated Risks During Pregnancy

Type of Lesion	Mechanism	Clinical Problems
Cyanotic	Low oxygen saturation Right-to-left shunt	Fetal loss, IUGR Systemic emboli
Shunt (left-to-right)	Right-to-left shunt with strain Right-sided volume overload Pulmonary hypertension High-velocity shunt	Paradoxical emboli Decreased reserve/failure Pulmonary artery rupture Endocarditis risk
Other (e.g., stenoses)	Decreased cardiac reserve Pulmonary hypertension High-velocity jet	CHF Pulmonary artery rupture Endocarditis risk

IUGR, intrauterine growth retardation; CHF, congestive heart failure.

and the exertional stress of delivery. Either or both of these stresses could cause symptoms of failure.

Because the actual effect on functional reserve can be difficult to assess on a resting echocardiogram, in situations where there is some doubt, I recommend exercise echocardiography both to assess the functional capacity compared with normal values and to see the effect of exercise on the hemodynamic parameters and ventricular function. Warning signs of potential difficulty include markedly reduced exercise capacity, reduced ventricular function with exercise, and dramatic deterioration in hemodynamic abnormalities.

Finally, the need for antibiotic prophylaxis during delivery needs to be assessed, with the usual risk factors of prosthetic materials in the heart, significant valvular regurgitation or stenosis, or a high-velocity shunt.

INSURABILITY AND CONGENITAL HEART DISEASE

In the past, patients with unoperated or operated congenital heart disease were virtually uninsurable when it came to obtaining life insurance. Fortunately, a task force addressed this issue and came up with recommendations that have alleviated the problem. However, patients with a cardiac history still may be denied insurance.

The guidelines include a classification of risk based on the degree of residual defects and physiological consequences of those effects. Although an echocardiographic examination is rarely performed solely to assess insurability, it is worthwhile to know the important parameters. These guidelines were developed before quantitative Doppler echocardiography, and so they are biased toward catheterization data. The hemodynamic evaluations, listed in Box 6–13, can now almost always be done with echocardiography. Note that there are additional clinical and electrocardiographic criteria that are not listed, including symptoms and rhythm disturbances.

BOX 6–13
ECHOCARDIOGRAPHIC HEMODYNAMIC EVALUATION FOR INSURABILITY

Pulmonic stenosis
  Peak gradient
Ductus arteriosus
  Ratio of total pulmonary flow to total systemic flow (Qp:Qs)
  Peak right ventricular pressure
Aortic stenosis
  Left ventricular size
  Left ventricular thickness
  Peak gradient
Atrial septal defect
  Qp:Qs
  Peak right ventricular pressure
Ventricular septal defect
  Qp:Qs
  Peak right ventricular pressure
Tetralogy of Fallot
  Qp:Qs
  Peak right ventricular pressure

FOLLOW-UP OF HEART DISEASE

For the patient with either an operated or unoperated congenital defect, echocardiography has become the cornerstone of outpatient follow-up. This group of patients is very diverse, and it is difficult to develop universal guidelines. As a general rule, though, the goal of the follow-up examination is similar to that of the second phase of the initial assessment, that is, after the diagnosis has been made and we proceed to the assessment of physiological severity. In the follow-up examination, the severity is compared with the previously determined level to assess trends.

The difference, however, is that there are certain problems that are known to develop in association with particular defects over the longer term that are not usually present at first. These problems are specific to each lesion and are highly variable. A few of the more common follow-up issues are discussed next and are summarized in Box 6–14.

Ventricular Septal Defect

The potential problems related to the follow-up of an isolated ventricular septal defect depend on the type of defect, when it

---

BOX 6–14
PARTICULAR FEATURES TO LOOK FOR IN FOLLOW-UP OF OPERATED PATIENTS

Ventricular septal defect
  Residual shunt
  Right ventricular peak systolic pressure
Ductus arteriosus
  Residual shunt
  Right ventricular peak systolic pressure
Atrial septal defect
  Residual shunt
  Right ventricular peak systolic pressure
  Right ventricular size and function
Coarctation of the aorta
  Residual coarctation
  Associated lesions (aortic, mitral, ventricular septal defect)
Atrioventricular septal defect
  Residual shunt
  Right ventricular peak systolic pressure
  Degree of mitral regurgitation
Tetralogy of Fallot
  Residual shunt
  Right ventricular peak systolic pressure
  Pulmonic stenosis/insufficiency
  Size of main pulmonary artery
Transposition of the great arteries
  Intra-atrial repair
    Caval obstruction
    Right (systemic) ventricular function
  Arterial switch
    Stenosis of main pulmonary artery

---

was repaired, and whether there are known residua. The simplest case is a perimembranous or supracristal ventricular septal defect that has been repaired in childhood with no known residua. We would normally look for residual ventricular septal flow, and estimate right ventricular pressures. We would also look for aortic insufficiency.

The case of a small, restrictive defect is similar, with assessment of the right ventricular function, degree of shunt, and restriction.

For ventricular septal defects of the atrioventricular septal defect type, it is also important to evaluate the degree of leakage of the mitral valve caused by clefts and abnormalities of chordal insertion.

Patent Ductus Arteriosus

Of all of the congenital defect repairs, closure of patent ductus arteriosus comes closest to a "perfect" repair. In most cases, patients with repaired ductus arteriosus have completely normal cardiac function and prognosis. The exceptions are rare and can be detected by echocardiography.

There may be a small chance of residual shunt, especially if the ductus was simply ligated. This can be detected in the same way as a native ductus and is in the same location (see Fig. 6–16). If a shunt is detected, the physiological evaluation is the same as for a native ductus; key factors are the pressure gradient across the shunt and any evidence for volume overload, such as enlargement of the left atrium and possibly the left ventricle. If the ductus was divided at the time of closure, the chance of a residual shunt is dramatically reduced.

The other possible residual problem related to closure of a patent ductus arteriosus is the development of pulmonary vascular disease. The risk of this occurring is related to the age of the patient at the time of repair, with later repair associated with greater risk, and the degree of shunt and pulmonary hypertension before repair. In general, if a follow-up echocardiogram after repair shows normal right-sided pressures, the risk of later development is probably nonexistent.

On the basis of these considerations, if a patient has a follow-up echocardiogram after closure of a patent ductus arteriosus and there is no evidence of a residual shunt and pulmonary hypertension, there is probably little chance of later development of these problems. Thus, further examinations may not be necessary.

Atrial Septal Defect

Repair of atrial septal defects is similar to that of ductus arteriosus in terms of being a "perfect" repair. Most patients have normal physiology and prognosis. Atrial arrhythmias may present problems for patients without residual defects but are not detectable by echocardiography, nor are there particular risk factors that are seen on the echocardiogram.

Otherwise, there is a small risk of residual defects and pulmonary vascular disease. As in the case of ductus arteriosus, residual defects can be detected by the same techniques as native atrial septal defects. If there are normal pulmonary pressures on an early examination, later development of pulmonary hypertension is unlikely. There is frequently a small residual shunt immediately after repair that may close over time.

Right ventricular size does not return to normal in a significant proportion of those operated on late in childhood or later.

Coarctation of the Aorta

There are three significant issues in the follow-up of the patient with repaired coarctation of the aorta, two of which can be assessed echocardiographically. The first issue is the presence or absence of residual coarctation. The chance of this developing is related to the age of the patient at the time of repair and the type of repair. Factors related to a higher risk of recurrence are early repair and an end-to-end repair. The major cause of recurrence is scarring and slower or absent growth of the repair site and adjacent tissues relative to the growth of the child. This means that if the patient has reached adulthood and does not have a gradient, it is unlikely to develop later.

Two technical points are worth mentioning in the follow-up of repaired coarctation (Fig. 6–22). First, in the assessment of coarctation gradients, the velocity proximal to the repair site is frequently significant, and using the "simplified" Bernoulli equation, with only the velocity through the narrowing, will result in a falsely high gradient estimate. Second, there is frequently a slight funnel shape to the area around the repair, which leads to a flow disturbance, causing a "spike" in the flow profile. The peak velocity in this case does not reflect a true gradient and will overestimate the peak gradient. Calculation of the mean gradient will yield correct values, however.

The second issue that can be assessed echocardiographically is the presence of any residual associated defects. The most common associated defects are bicuspid aortic valve, ventricular septal defect, and mitral regurgitation. These should be looked for in follow-up examinations.

The third issue for patients being evaluated after coarctation repair is the development of systemic hypertension. This is a lifelong risk, which is increased with later age at time of repair and cannot be assessed echocardiographically.

Atrioventricular Septal Defect

Repair of an atrioventricular septal defect is never perfect. In addition to the expected issues of whether there is a residual shunt through the repairs of the ventricular and atrial portions of the defect, there is always some degree of residual mitral regurgitation even after successful repair of the cleft mitral valve.

Consequently, in follow-up, in addition to the expected areas of focus on the presence or absence of residual atrial and ventricular level shunts and pulmonary vascular disease, the degree of mitral regurgitation should always be assessed.

Tetralogy of Fallot

The findings and areas of focus after repair of tetralogy of Fallot depend on the

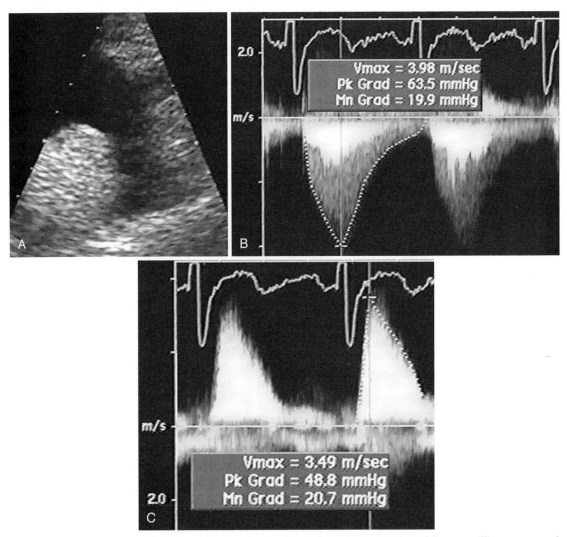

Figure 6–22. Follow-up images from a patient with previous repair of a coarctation of the aorta. The suprasternal image suggests that there is some narrowing in the area of the repair (A), and there is an acceleration of flow with a high peak velocity (B). This peak velocity may overestimate the peak gradient, although the mean gradient is more reliable. Note the visible proximal flow velocity on this continuous-wave Doppler recording. Finally, this patient also has aortic stenosis, of significant degree, as shown by a continuous-wave Doppler recording through the aortic valve (C).

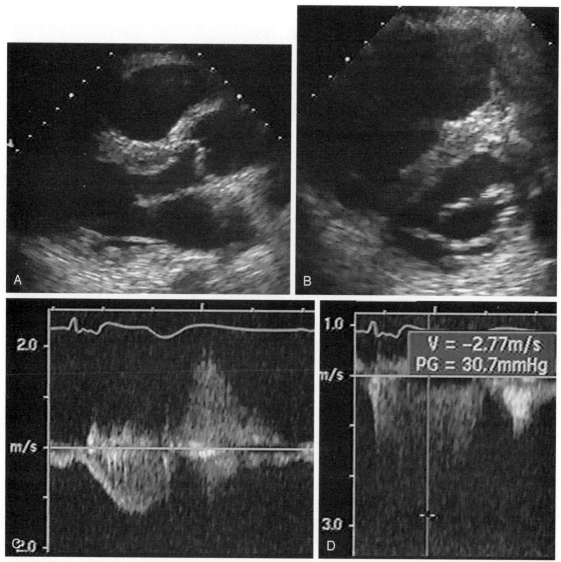

Figure 6–23. Images from a patient who had previous repair of tetralogy of Fallot. The parasternal long-axis images show that there is enlargement and, therefore, volume overload of the right ventricle as well as the exaggerated override of the aorta, even after repair *(A)*. The right ventricular enlargement is also apparent in the short-axis view *(B)*. Doppler through the pulmonic valve shows no acceleration for forward flow, but there is unrestricted reverse flow, which rapidly decays to baseline *(C)*. This indicates severe pulmonary insufficiency. There is mild elevation of the right ventricular peak systolic pressure because of increased flow, as evidenced by the tricuspid insufficiency velocity *(D)*.

type of repair. Patients without hypoplasia of the pulmonary outflow who have had primarily valvular pulmonic stenosis may have had a pulmonary valvotomy and retain their native outflow tract. Those with a hypoplastic outflow tract may have had either a procedure widening the outflow using a patch, which is usually pericardial, or replacement with a pulmonary homograft.

For the patients who have had a pulmonary valvotomy, the results are often very good, although some of these patients have severe pulmonic insufficiency, with resulting serious right ventricular enlargement (Fig. 6–23). These patients should be examined for residual ventricular septal defect as well as residual pulmonic stenosis or insufficiency. It is rare for these patients to have either peripheral pulmonic stenosis or pulmonary vascular disease, but both should be checked for by estimating pulmonary pressures.

The hemodynamic results with a pulmonary homograft are frequently quite good, although the long-term follow-up of pulmonary homografts is not known. The major difference is that these patients are more likely to have peripheral pulmonic stenosis because they had a hypoplastic pulmonary artery to begin with, and this may raise the pressure in the main pulmonary artery and right ventricle.

Finally, patients who have had patch en-largement of the right ventricular outflow are at risk for peripheral pulmonic stenosis, similar to the patient with a pulmonary homograft, but with two additional concerns. First, these patients always have significant pulmonic insufficiency, which is sometimes severe. Second, these patients are subject to aneurysm of the right ventricular outflow patch, especially if there is elevation of right ventricular pressure.

Transposition of the Great Arteries

The long-term problems that can be associated with a repaired transposition of the great arteries depend on the type of repair. We encounter three types of repairs in this age group. The oldest patients have some type of intra-atrial repair, either of the Mustard or Senning type. In addition to differences in the geometry of these two repairs (Figs. 6–24 to 6–26), there is a difference in the material used to construct the new channels for blood. In the Mustard repair, the baffle is constructed from pericardium or Dacron, whereas with Senning repair the atrial wall itself is used. This may explain why the Mustard procedure is more subject to stenosis of the venous inflow, which is rare in the Senning repair. It may be due to scarring of the material of the baffle as well as different geometry. Stenosis can be assessed by examining the superior and infe-

Figure 6–24. Diagram illustrating the differences in appearance between a Mustard (upper) and Senning (lower) operation for transposition of the great arteries. The left images are in the pediatric orientation, and the right images are in the adult orientation. These drawings are derived from the images in Figures 6–25 and 6–26. (IVC, inferior vena cava; RV, right ventricle; LV, left ventricle.)

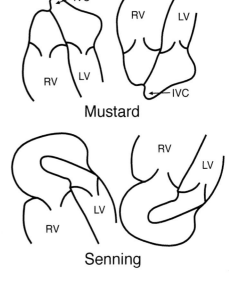

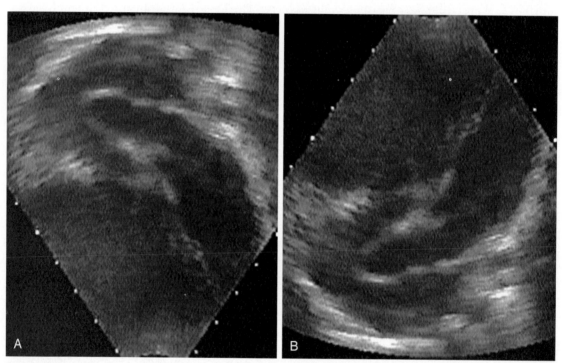

Figure 6–25. Apical four-chamber views in the pediatric *(A)* and adult *(B)* orientation from a child with transposition of the great arteries and Senning repair. Note the appearance of a "channel" going from the mitral valve toward the inferior vena cava and a "dogleg" from the tricuspid valve toward the pulmonary veins.

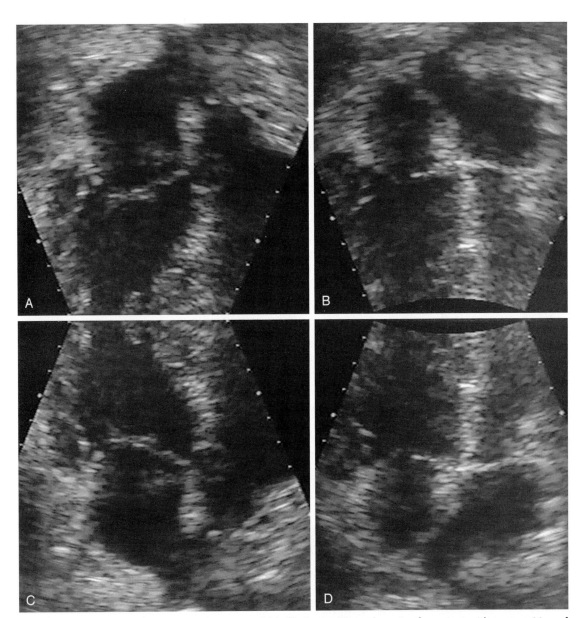

Figure 6–26. These images illustrate the intra-atrial baffle in the Mustard repair of a patient with transposition of the great arteries. The images are obtained in the apical four-chamber orientation, showing the channel leading blood from the pulmonary veins to the right (systemic) ventricle (*A*, pediatric orientation; *C*, adult orientation). With a slight difference in angulation, it is possible to see the channel leading blood from the vena cava to the left (pulmonary) ventricle (*B*, pediatric orientation; *D*, adult orientation). Note that the right ventricle is large and hypertrophic.

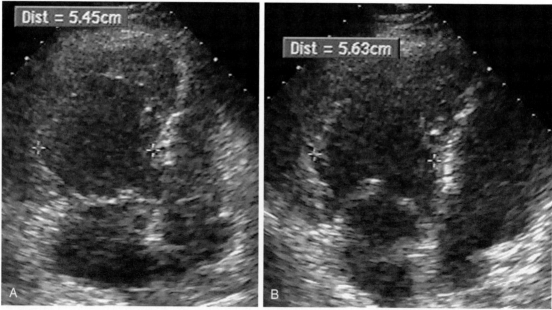

Figure 6–27. These images show the very poor right (systemic) ventricular function in a patient with transposition of the great arteries, Mustard repair, and symptoms of systemic ventricular failure. Both images are four-chamber apical views in the adult orientation. There is very little difference between the right ventricular dimensions in systole *(A)* and diastole *(B)*.

rior vena cava flow into the atria using pulsed Doppler.

Both repairs can lead to long-term right ventricular failure, however, and right ventricular function should be assessed in all these patients on a regular basis (Fig. 6–27). Right ventricular function generally appears lower in these patients than in normal individuals because of the differences in geometry of the right ventricle, which generally looks dilated (Fig. 6–28). Also, calculations of right ventricular ejection fraction generally yield lower values than normal for the left ventricle.

The arterial switch procedure has none of these problems, but, depending on the details of the geometry of the repair, there may be supravalvular pulmonary stenosis in up to 30% of patients or, occasionally, problems with the coronary arteries.

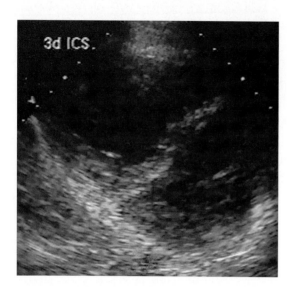

Figure 6–28. The right ventricle always looks dilated and hypertrophic when the patient has transposition of the great arteries and an intra-atrial baffle procedure, as demonstrated in this parasternal short-axis image from an asymptomatic patient with a Mustard repair.

Echocardiographic Planes

For all types of clinical imaging, there are standard views and standard orientations to present them. This facilitates interpretation of the images by those who did not perform the examination themselves. The main standard echocardiographic cross-sections, or views, were discussed in Chapter 1 and are shown in Figure A–1. These are oriented with respect to the left ventricle as if it were a cylinder, with the short-axis view cutting across the short axis of the cylinder and two views oriented along the long axis of the cylinder. These two views along the long axis of the ventricle are the four-chamber view, which includes the right ventricle, and the long-axis view, which includes the left ventricular outflow. All other standard views are related to these main views. Each of these views can be obtained from at least two different echocardiographic windows (Fig. A–2; see also Fig. 1–19).

Even with the standard views, there can be at least eight different orientations to present a given view! The orientations are easily understood if we label a piece of paper with a different number (e.g., 1, 2, 3, 4) along each edge. We can orient the paper with any one of the numbers at the top, so that makes four different orientations. A mirror image of the page is represented by the other side, which also clearly has four edges, and hence we have eight possible orientations (Fig. A–3). Fortunately, the actual orientations used are limited by the conventions used in anatomy and other imaging techniques in medicine.

Naming Principles

The naming conventions are best understood by considering the three major anatomic planes: coronal, sagittal, and transverse (Fig. A–4). The coronal planes divide the body front to back and are often called the frontal planes for that reason, whereas the sagittal planes divide the body right from left. The transverse planes divide the body top from bottom and are also called the cross-sectional planes.

Each of these planes can have at least eight orientations, as noted previously. The convention for the frontal planes is to present them as you would see them when face to face with the standing patient. This means that cephalad (toward the head) is at the top of the image, and the right of the patient is on the left of the image, just as if you were looking directly at the patient.

The sagittal images are oriented as if you are at the patient's left, with the patient standing. Anterior is to the left, and the patient's head is at the top of the image.

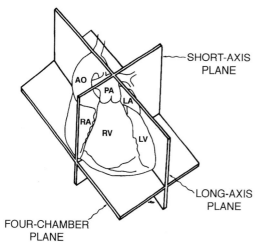

Figure A–1. The three major planes are oriented with respect to the left ventricle (LV) as if it were a cylinder. The short-axis plane crosses the cylinder transversely, whereas the long-axis and four-chamber planes are oriented along the long axis of the left ventricle, but the long-axis view includes the left ventricular outflow. (AO, aorta; PA, pulmonary artery; RA, right atrium; LA, left atrium; RV, right ventricle.) (From Henry WL, DeMaria A, Gramiak R, et al. Report of the American Society of Echocardiography Committee on nomenclature and standards in two-dimensional echocardiography. Circulation 1980; 62(2):212–215.)

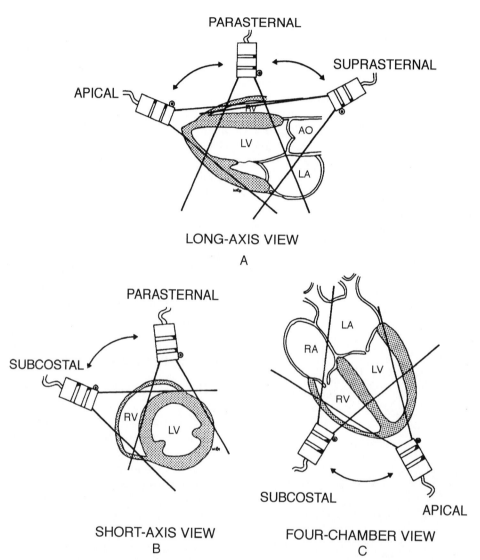

Figure A–2. A–C, Each of the three main views can be obtained from at least two different echocardiographic windows, although in a different orientation. (RV, right ventricle; LV, left ventricle; AO, aorta; LA, left atrium; RA, right atrium.) (From Henry WL, DeMaria A, Gramiak R, et al. Report of the American Society of Echocardiography Committee on nomenclature and standards in two-dimensional echocardiography. Circulation 1980; 62(2):212–215.)

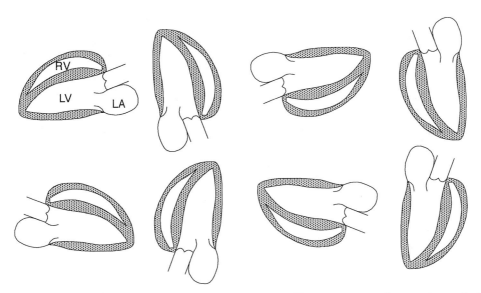

Figure A–3. A given view can be oriented in many arbitrary ways. The top views are the same long-axis view, just rotated clockwise 90 degrees. This corresponds to what would happen if we had a paper copy of the image and rotated it 90 degrees. The lower views are mirror images of the top views, illustrating that they are, in fact, different as well. (RV, right ventricle; LV, left ventricle; LA, left atrium.)

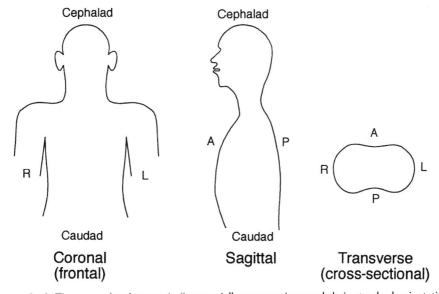

Figure A–4. These are the three main "anatomic" cross-sections and their standard orientations.

For the transverse planes, the convention is that they are oriented as if you were at the foot of the bed of the supine patient, looking toward the head. That means that the top of the image is anterior, or ventral, and the right of the patient is on the left of the image.

Challenges in Echocardiography

All of these standards work well for images that are oriented along the major planes, such as coronal, sagittal, and transverse. What happens when we are imaging in a plane that is between two of the major planes? As expected, the results can be chaotic. Although none of the major echocardiographic imaging planes coincides with the anatomic planes and, therefore, each has two different possible "standard orientations," the potential chaos this could cause has been limited mostly to the subcostal and apical four-chamber views.

The subcostal view is directed at an angle somewhere between the transverse and coronal cross-sections (Fig. A–5). If we were to orient it as if it were a transverse section, we would put anterior at the top and the patient's right to the left of the image. This is the convention used in adult cardiology and is sometimes referred to as "vertex-up" because the origin of the sector image is at the top of the image. If we were to consider the subcostal four-chamber view to be closer

to the coronal plane, we would orient it so that cephalad is at the top of the image and the left of the image would be the patient's right. This is merely a vertically flipped version of the "adult" view, and all modern ultrasound machines allow the operator to perform this transformation by changing some options. This is the orientation used in pediatric cardiology and is sometimes referred to as "vertex-down."

An additional problem with echocardiography resulted from the hardware limitations of ultrasound machines. The display hardware could be fairly easily modified to allow "flipping" of the image on the vertical or horizontal axes, or both, but rotation of the image was much more difficult. This meant that it was possible to create a "mirror image," exchanging right and left on the image, or present the image with the sector vertex at the top or the bottom of the image. Presentation with the vertex to the right or left or any intermediate angle was much more difficult and usually not done.

The apical four-chamber views are affected by both this hardware limitation and the ambiguity caused by oblique planes. The problem is that the transducer is located toward the patient's left (assuming levocardia), and neither the vertex-up nor vertex-down orientation corresponds to anatomic orientations because they would be displaying the patient's left as at the top or bottom of the image, respectively. Because the hardware could present the apex at the top or the bottom of the screen, for adult orientations, this means that the apex of the heart is at the top of the screen and that the left ventricle is on the right of the image. For pediatric orientations, it means that the apex of the heart is downward and the left ventricle is on the right of the image as well (Fig. A–6). Thus, the subcostal and apical four-chamber views in either adult or pediatric cardiology can be rotated to match the other view.

The problems in reconciling the other echocardiographic views with standard imaging views were generally not as great. This can be easily seen if we consider the parasternal long-axis view as a sagittal view (Fig. A–7). If we were to adhere to the standard in other imaging techniques, we

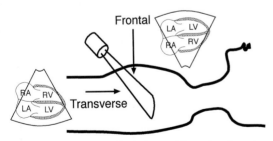

Figure A–5. Because the subcostal four-chamber view is oblique, it can be considered a variant of the cross-sectional views (left) or the frontal views (top). The net effect is to flip the view along the horizontal axis. The "frontal" view is used in pediatric cardiology, whereas the "cross-sectional" view is used in adult cardiology. (RA, right atrium; LA, left atrium; RV, right ventricle; LV, left ventricle.)

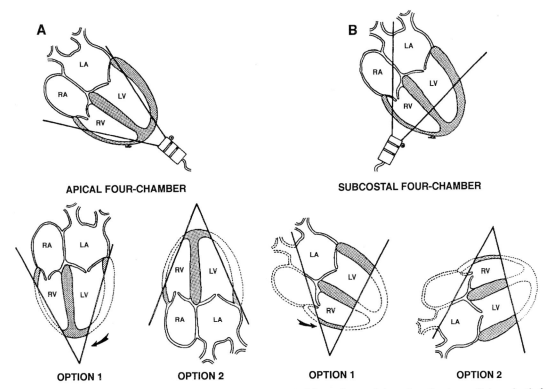

A

B

APICAL FOUR-CHAMBER

SUBCOSTAL FOUR-CHAMBER

OPTION 1   **OPTION 2**   **OPTION 1**   **OPTION 2**

Figure A–6. *A* and *B,* The four-chamber views are oriented differently in adult and pediatric cardiology, both for the subcostal and apical views. The "vertex down" versions, labeled "Option 1," are preferred in pediatric cardiology, whereas the "vertex up" versions are preferred in adult cardiology. (LA, left atrium; RA, right atrium; LV, left ventricle; RV, right ventricle.) (From Henry WL, DeMaria A, Gramiak R, et al. Report of the American Society of Echocardiography Committee on nomenclature and standards in two-dimensional echocardiography. Circulation 1980; 62(2):212–215.)

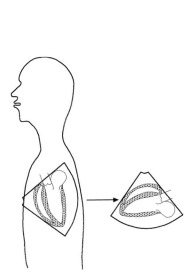

Figure A–7. Because of hardware limitations, the standard orientation of the parasternal views, with the vertex of the sector to the left, was not possible. As a compromise, the images were rotated 90 degrees to the right for the standard views.

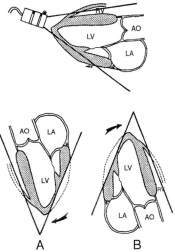

A   **B**

Figure A–8. The orientation of the apical long-axis views differs in adult and pediatric cardiology. In pediatric cardiology, it is presented vertex down (left lower), whereas in adult cardiology, the vertex is up (right lower). (LV, left ventricle; RV, right ventricle; LA, left atrium; AO, aorta.) (From Henry WL, DeMaria A, Gramiak R, et al. Report of the American Society of Echocardiography Committee on nomenclature and standards in two-dimensional echocardiography. Circulation 1980; 62(2):212–215.)

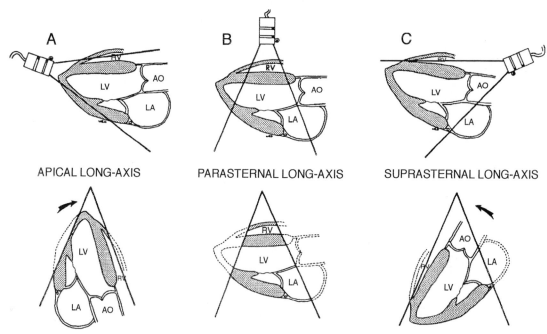

Figure A–9. *A–C,* Because of the limitations in display hardware, the orientation of the image of a given view varies depending on the echocardiographic window. (RV, right ventricle; LV, left ventricle; AO, aorta; LA, left atrium.) (From Henry WL, DeMaria A, Gramiak R, et al. Report of the American Society of Echocardiography Committee on nomenclature and standards in two-dimensional echocardiography. Circulation 1980; 62(2):212–215.)

would need to put the vertex of the image to the left, which was difficult to do. The compromise was to rotate the image by a one-quarter turn in the clockwise direction as if the patient were supine. This means that the top of the image is anterior and the right is cephalad (toward the patient's head). For the apical long-axis images, the adult orientation has the vertex at the top of the image and the aortic valve to the right. The pediatric orientations of the long-axis view are with the parasternal views presented identically to the adult views,

whereas the apical view is with the apex down and the aortic valve to the left (Fig. A–8).

For the parasternal views, the short axis is always oriented as if it is a transverse view of the body. This means that anterior should be at the top of the image and the right of the patient is on the left of the image. Because of the limitations of the display hardware, the orientation of even these views changes when the access window changes, as shown for the long-axis view in Figure A–9.

Abnormal Position and Connection of Cardiac Structures

Abnormal position and connection of the cardiac structures can cause a great deal of confusion. Not only are the familiar echocardiographic views and orientations not available from the standard windows, but the nomenclature for the various malpositions is not always clear, and often applied inconsistently.

Fortunately, for most situations, the critical clinical decisions are based on the physiology and connections, which is the reason for the emphasis in Chapter 2. The details of position and orientation can have significance for surgical approach, however, and also for the chance of associated lesions. For this reason, such abnormalities are worth discussion here.

A common approach to these abnormalities is to "follow the blood flow," starting with the systemic venous connections and atria and progressing to the great vessels (Anderson et al, 1983). This has a logical appeal and allows for detailed specification of even the most complex congenital abnormalities. In my opinion, however, this approach starts with the abnormalities that are of least frequent clinical significance and most confusing (i.e., abnormalities of visceral situs).

Therefore, we will take an approach emphasizing echocardiographic and clinical importance. Because the position of the heart in the chest influences the entire exam, this is the first subject discussed, followed by discussion of the position of the great arteries and the position of the atria.

Before we begin this discussion, it is worth recalling that the cardiac structures have anatomic names that *imply* their location in a certain orientation, such as right ventricle, left atrium, and so on. This is not the case, and these names should be considered anatomic names only, irrespective of location or connections. Similarly, the anatomic name is not determined by the physiological function of a structure. The right ventricle is still the right ventricle whether it is on the right or left of the patient and whether it carries oxygenated or unoxygenated blood. Also, there is much confusion with terms that refer to position or orientation rather than connections.

Abnormal Cardiac Position

The heart is normally located predominantly in the left side of the chest. Hence, if the heart is located in the right half of the chest (dextrocardia) or even in the midline (mesocardia), this is an abnormal position.

Even in the most abnormal case, which is dextrocardia, the orientation of the heart can be variable, and the term dextrocardia gives no hint as to the orientation. Fortunately, there are only three main variants, which can be distinguished by the relative position of the right and left ventricles and the apex of the heart. In the normal situation (levocardia), the apex of the heart points to the left, the right ventricle is anterior (not on the right!), and the left ventricle is posterior. It can be helpful to think of the right ventricle as oriented like the right hand held over the heart. The thumb is the main pulmonary artery, and the fingers point toward the apex (Fig. B–1, normal).

The simplest case is when the heart is

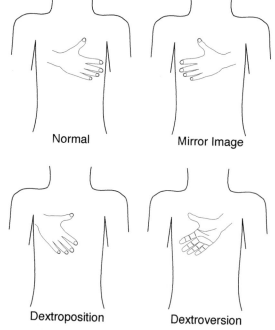

Normal   Mirror Image

Dextroposition   Dextroversion

Figure B–1. We can illustrate some of the malpositions of the heart by using the right hand to symbolize the right ventricle. The normal position is with the fingers (apex) pointed to the left, with the main part of the ventricle in the mid to left side of the chest. In dextroposition, the orientation is the same, but the heart is shifted into the right side of the chest. In dextroversion, the heart is rotated, so that the apex is pointed to the right. In mirror-image dextrocardia, it is as though there were a left hand, pointed to the left.

oriented normally but is shifted to the right. It is as though the right hand is kept in the same orientation but just moved over the right chest. This is probably most clearly termed dextroposition (see Fig. B–1, dextroposition). It may be caused by hypoplasia of the right lung or overinflation of the left lung. In this case, the apical views can often be best obtained from the subxiphoid position and the parasternal views obtained from the right parasternal position.

The next easiest situation to understand is mirror-image dextrocardia. In this case, everything is a mirror image of the normal situation. The apex points toward the right, and the right ventricle is anterior and best represented by a left hand on the right chest (see Fig. B–1, mirror image). This is relatively uncommon, occurring primarily in Kartagener's syndrome and other rare disorders.

The final variant is more common than mirror-image dextrocardia but also more confusing. In this case, the apex of the heart can be considered to have rotated around the base until it is pointed to the right. As a result, the right ventricle is posterior, and the representation of the right ventricle would be a right hand rotated so that the fingers point to the right and the palm is facing forward (see Fig. B–1, dextroversion). This type of dextrocardia is best termed dextroversion, or dextrorotation. It is also commonly associated with many other significant abnormalities and atrial isomerism, which is discussed further later (see Abnormal Position and Connection of the Atria). An intermediate form is when the apex of the heart is partially "rotated" so that it points toward the midline. This is usually associated with a midline position of the heart and is referred to as mesocardia. It is also usually associated with significant heart defects.

Abnormal Orientation and Connection of the Great Arteries

The normal orientation of the great arteries is such that the aorta originates posterior to the pulmonary artery from the left ventricle and loops to the left of the patient, coursing down the left side of the spinal column. The pulmonary artery originates anteriorly from the right ventricle, coursing posteriorly and to the left of the aorta. The right pulmonary artery actually ends up coursing posteriorly to the aorta. This normal positioning is sometimes called *l-normal* because the aorta is to the left of the pulmonary artery at its origin, and the orientation of the pulmonary artery and aorta in the anteroposterior direction is normal. The "l" stands for "levo," or left. The term l-normal refers to position, however, not to connections. Caveat lector!

In mirror-image dextrocardia the right-left orientation is reversed, although everything else is the same. This means that the aorta is to the right and posterior to the pulmonary artery at its origin. This orientation is sometimes called *d-normal*, with the "d" standing for "dextro," or right. Again, d-normal refers to positioning only, and in the case described the connections are normal.

The relationship of the great arteries can be normal or inverted. That is, the aorta can originate anteriorly or posteriorly. If the aorta originates anteriorly and to the right of the pulmonary artery, the position is called *d-transposition*. The most important issue physiologically is which ventricle each great artery is connected to. This can be normal, or inverted, or both arteries may come from the same ventricle. A few examples can help clarify this distinction.

In the most common form of transposition of the great arteries (also called complete transposition of the great arteries), the connections of the great arteries are inverted, but the position and connections of the heart are otherwise unchanged. This can also be called d-transposition because the aorta originated anterior to and to the right of the pulmonary artery.

In the case of dextroversion of the heart, if the aorta is still connected to the left ventricle, its origin will become anterior to the origin of the pulmonary artery. Whether it is to the right or the left of the pulmonary artery depends on other details of anatomy and rotation. So, it may be d-transposition, l-transposition, or a-transposition, in which "a" indicates that the aorta is directly anterior, neither right nor left. Note that because this terminology depends on relative position rather than connections, this normal connection is labeled "transposition." This also illustrates that d-transposition should not be used as a synonym for complete transposition of the great arteries.

Abnormal Position and Connection of the Atria

We frequently distinguish the atria based on the venous and ventricular connection, but this will obviously not work in the case of abnormal connections. The anatomist or pathologist can distinguish the atria based on the morphology of the atrial appendages; the left atrial appendage is long and thin, whereas the right atrial appendage is both broad based and short. These details can be difficult to determine on a transthoracic

echocardiographic examination and possibly even on transesophageal echocardiograms.

For these reasons, two other methods are commonly used. Both are based on the fact that the configuration of the atria usually follows the configuration of the other visceral organs. This means that if in a given patient the positions of the right and left atria are reversed, such as in mirror-image dextrocardia, the positions of the anatomic right and left lungs are also reversed. More surprisingly, a person can have two anatomic left atria, each a mirror image of the other, and then will have two left lungs. This is not as confusing when one remembers that the terms "right" and "left," in this context, have nothing to do with the right and left sides of the patient and are only anatomic terms.

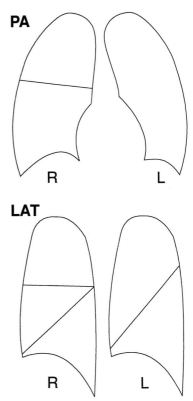

Figure B–2. The two lungs have different morphology. On the posteroanterior (PA) projection, the right (R) lung has a horizontal fissure, which is often visible between the upper and other two lobes. The left (L) lung has only a diagonal fissure, which is not visible on this view but is illustrated below in the lateral (LAT) projection. Because the two lungs are superimposed on the lateral projection, it is not possible to distinguish the two lungs on that view.

This means that if we can determine the configuration of each of the lungs, we can deduce the configuration of the atria. We cannot easily see the configuration of the lungs on echocardiography, but we can use a plain chest x-ray film to help us. The radiographic features of lung morphology that we can easily see have to do with the fissures and the bronchi.

The right lung has three lobes, imaginatively called upper, lower, and middle. The divisions between the lobes are called fissures, and the fissure between the upper and middle lobe is oriented horizontally and is, therefore, often visible end-on in the posteroanterior (PA) (for the direction of the x-ray beam) chest x-ray film as a horizontal line (Fig. B–2). The left lung has only two lobes, the upper and lower, and the fissure runs diagonally downward and is, therefore, not visible on the PA chest film.

The other finding has to do with the bronchial morphology (Fig. B–3). Several features distinguish the right and left bronchi. The left main bronchus is directed at a wider angle relative to the trachea and has a longer distance to its first branch. The

right main bronchus has a narrower angle relative to the trachea, is shorter overall, and has a shorter stretch to its first main branch. These details can often be made more visible on the PA film by viewing the film at an angle, which enhances the contrast.

Both of these techniques rely on the availability of a chest film. The echocardiographic techniques rely on the venous connections, which are also related to the atrial morphology but not as closely (Fig. B–4). In brief, a right atrium usually has an inferior vena cava attached to it, even if it is on the left. This is illustrated in Figure B–4. When there is duplication of the right atria, so that the patient has two right atria, the condition is called right atrial isomerism and is usually associated with other significant anomalies. In this situation, the inferior vena cava and the aorta are often located on the same side of the spine, either right or left, and the inferior vena cava is anterior. When there is left atrial isomerism, there is frequently interruption of the inferior vena cava, and the connection is via an azygos or hemiazygos vein. This is

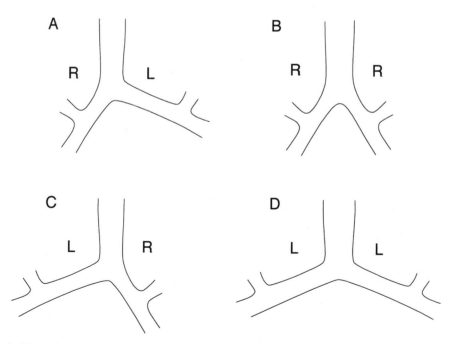

Figure B–3. The right (R) and left (L) bronchi are different in configuration (A). The right is more "in line" with the trachea, and the first branch point occurs earlier. The left takes off at a wider angle and has a longer distance to the first branch point. It is possible to have a mirror-image configuration (C), two right bronchi (B), or two left bronchi (D).

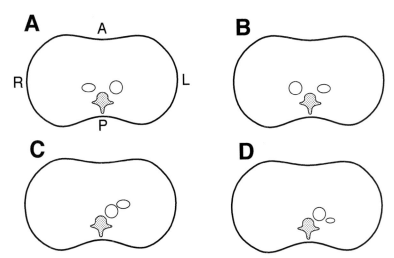

Figure B–4. The atrial morphology may often be inferred from the vessels on the abdomen, as seen in this schematic of a cross-sectional image. The normal situation *(A)* is that the aorta (circle) is on the left of the spine and the inferior vena cava (IVC, oval shape) is on the right. The mirror-image configuration is opposite *(B)*. If there are two right atria, the aorta and inferior vena cava (IVC) are often on the same side, which can be either right or left, with the IVC anterior *(C)*. If there are two left atria, the IVC is often interrupted, and the venous drainage from the lower half of the body is through the azygos or hemiazygos vein, which is smaller and posterior to the aorta *(D)*.

smaller than an inferior vena cava and is located posterior to the aorta.

Another consequence of this connection between atrial and visceral anatomy is the relationship between atrial isomerism and asplenia/polysplenia syndromes. Patients who have two morphological left atria tend to have polysplenia because the spleen, which is located on the left, is duplicated as well. Patients with right atrial isomerism tend to have asplenia for the converse reason. Patients with asplenia are more susceptible to certain types of infections, such as pneumococcal sepsis.

Because this is a practical text rather than a reference book, the emphasis in this bibliography is on books that I have actually used, articles that I have found to illustrate a given point particularly well, and relevant articles that I have written. As such, it is somewhat idiosyncratic. This is not a complete list, nor does it cover all of the topics in this book. I have also included some comments on each of the entries. I have listed the most recently available edition, even when I have used an older one.

General

Fink BW. Congenital Heart Disease. St. Louis, MO, Mosby Year Book, 1991.
This small paperback is a very good, basic, although somewhat dated introduction to congenital heart disease. It is practically oriented and succeeds in making complex concepts easier to understand.

Hatle L, Angelsen BAJ. Doppler Ultrasound in Cardiology: Physical Principles and Clinical Applications. Philadelphia, Lea & Febiger, 1993.
Excellent overview of the principles in clinical application of Doppler echocardiography, covering both acquired and congenital heart disease.

Henry WL, DeMaria A, Gramiak R, et al. Report of the American Society of Echocardiography Committee on nomenclature and standards in two-dimensional echocardiography. Circulation 1980;62(2):212–215.
Standards for echocardiographic image orientation.

Perloff JK. The Clinical Recognition of Congenital Heart Disease. Philadelphia, WB Saunders, 1994.
This is an excellent book with good illustrations. Its clinical orientation is its strength.

Morphology/Embryology

Anderson RH, Becker AE, Lucchese FE, et al. Morphology of Congenital Heart Disease. Baltimore, MD, University Park Press, 1983.
This small book is a good introduction to segmental analysis, as done by Anderson. I have found it to be a valuable source for the details of morphology of the ventricles, septa, and valves in many different abnormalities.

Langman J. Medical Embryology. Baltimore, MD, Williams & Wilkins, 1981.
This is an excellent general embryology textbook, with extensive sections on congenital heart defects.

Fetus/Neonate/Child

Allan LD. Manual of Fetal Echocardiology. Norwell, MA, Kluwer Academic, 1986.
This early book is a good introduction to the topic. I do not, however, agree with the author's suggestion that a four-chamber view is adequate for screening.

Copel JA, Friedman AH, Kleinman CS. Management of fetal arrhythmias. Obstet Gynecol Clin North Am 1997;24(1):201–211.
This review article is a good starting point for understanding fetal arrhythmias and their treatment.

Emmanouilides GC, Riemenschneider TA, Allen HD, Gutgesell HP, eds. Moss and Adams' Heart Disease in Infants, Children and Adolescents: Including the Fetus and Young Adult, 5th ed. Baltimore, MD, Williams & Wilkins, 1994.
This multiauthor book is most useful as a reference book. There is necessarily less emphasis on the clinical approach and differential diagnosis, but this is still a book I use for reference.

Gembruch U, Shi C, Smrcek JM. Biometry of the fetal heart between 10 and 17 weeks of gestation. Fetal Diagn Ther 2000;15(1):20–31.
Extends measurements to earlier gestational ages.

Park MK. Pediatric Cardiology for Practitioners. St. Louis, MO, Mosby-Year Book, 1995.
This is a practically oriented book but somewhat sparse in style. It falls somewhere between Perloff's and Fink's works in terms of detail and illustrations.

Sahn DJ, Lange LW, Allen HD, et al. Quantitative real-time cross-sectional echocardiography in the developing human fetus and newborn. Circulation 1980; 62(3):588–597.
Normal values for cardiac measurements.

St. John Sutton MG, Gewitz MH, Shah B, et al. Quantitative assessment of growth and function of the cardiac chambers in the normal human fetus: a prospective longitudinal echocardiographic study. Circulation 1984;69(4):645–654.
Emphasizes that the ratio of sizes remains constant.

Adult

Corrado D, Basso C, Schiavon M, Thiene G. Screening for hypertrophic cardiomyopathy in young athletes. N Engl J Med 1988;339(6):364–369.
Interesting study from Italy, suggesting that a comprehensive and mandatory pre-athletic screening program can reduce deaths due to hypertrophic cardiomyopathy.

Maron BJ, Thompson PD, Puffer JC, et al. Cardiovascular preparticipation screening of competitive athletes: A statement for health professionals from the Sudden Death Committee (Clinical Cardiology) and Congenital Defects Committee (Cardiovascular Disease in the Young), American Heart Association. Circulation 1996;94(4):850–856.
This article presents committee recommendations regarding preparticipation examinations, which did not recommend routine echocardiography. It is a useful reference and review. See also the addendum (Circulation 1998;997:2294).

Perloff JK, Child JS. Congenital Heart Disease in Adults. Philadelphia, WB Saunders, 1998.
This is a good overview, best used as an introduction to this complex topic. Like Perloff's other book, its strength is its clinical orientation.

Skorton DJ, Garson A Jr, eds. Congenital heart disease in adolescents and adults. Cardiol Clin North Am 1993;11(4).
This entire issue of Cardiology Clinics of North America was devoted to specific topics in this broad area, including particular issues related to specific defects and repairs as well as issues of pregnancy, choice of career, and insurance, among others.

Talner NS, McCue HM Jr, Graham TP, et al. Guidelines for insurability of patient with congenital heart disease. Circulation 1980;62(6):1419A–1424A.

This was an effort in good faith to try to create guidelines that insurance companies could use to stratify risk of patients with congenital heart disease. It appears that the actual usage of these guidelines has been spotty at best. See also the article on the subject in a special edition of the *Cardiology Clinics of North America,* listed above.

Selected Articles by the Author

Andersen S, Vik T, Linker DT. [Congenital heart diseases in Sor-Trondelag. Incidence, diagnosis, course and treatment]. Tidsskr Nor Laegeforen 1994; 114(1):29–32.

This article estimates the incidence of congenital heart disease at at least 10/1000, using centralized referral after screening pediatric examinations and modern echocardiographic techniques for diagnosis. The actual article is in Norwegian.

Linker DT, Rossvoll O, Chapman JV, Angelsen BAJ. Sensitivity and speed of colour Doppler flow mapping compared with continuous wave Doppler for the detection of ventricular septal defects. Br Heart J 1991;65:201–203.

This article demonstrates that the speed of color Doppler is not different from continuous-wave Doppler and both are subject to errors. The best results are with an integrated examination.

Tegnander E, Eik-Nes SH, Johansen OJ, Linker DT. Prenatal detection of heart defects at the routine fetal examination at 18 weeks in a non-selected population. Ultrasound Obstet Gynecol 1995;5(6): 372–380.

The major finding is that, by using a four-chamber view on a screening examination, only 40% of defects were detected prenatally.

Index